Women's Wisdom

Natural Wellness Strategies for the Menstrual Years

Laurel Alexander

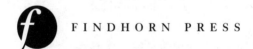

FINDHORN PRESS

Published in 2013 by Findhorn Press, Scotland

ISBN 978-1-84409-594-0

A CIP record for this title is available from the British Library.

Edited by Nicky Leach
Cover design and illustrations by Richard Crookes
Interior design by Damian Keenan
Printed and bound in the EU

1 2 3 4 5 6 7 8 9 17 16 15 14 13

Published by
Findhorn Press
117-121 High Street,
Forres IV36 1AB,
Scotland, UK

t +44 (0)1309 690582
f +44 (0)131 777 2711
e info@findhornpress.com
www.findhornpress.com

CONTENTS

Disclaimer

The information in this book is given in good faith and is neither
intended to diagnose any physical or mental condition nor to serve
as a substitute for informed medical advice or care.

Please contact your health professional for medical advice and
treatment. Neither author nor publisher can be held liable by any
person for any loss or damage whatsoever which may arise from the
use of this book or any of the information therein.

Prologue

I began this book the day my monthly bleed started in February 2012. It seemed the right time to begin a book on menstruation, as women are at their most creative a few days before, and the first couple of days into, their period. During this time, we can connect to our inner wisdom and draw out into daily living that which makes our lives authentic.

For a while, I am your guide for your menstrual journey. For the next few moments, let me share my journey with you.

I feel sad for the emptiness of my first blood. My mother wasn't present. My sister and stepfather told me of the practicalities of what would happen. It was a sterile exercise, and I entered womanhood with fear.

When I was a teenager, my period pains were horrendous. I recall lying in the sickroom at secondary school until I could stand it no longer and went home. I then threw up on the bus, much to the consternation of my fellow passengers.

We didn't have enough money for sanitary pads, so I was given cotton wool to soak up the blood. You can imagine the uncomfortable stickiness! My hand-me-down underpants (from my older sister) bulged with pad and cotton wool, and I remember the shame when it came to PE lessons. Another thing I remember was sanitary belts, which went around the waist with a hook front and back that linked with the loops on the sanitary pads. These have been around since the 19th century. Mine was a tad more modern than that—barely.

As I grew into womanhood, I was finally in charge of my own sanitary protection, thank heavens. I tried using tampons, but they made me physically sick to insert. Since then, I have found out that my vagina is very small. Pap smears were always painful until a kind nurse mentioned that I should always ask for the instruments suitable for "virgins."

My emotions during the week before my period used to be dreadful—full of anger. When I was younger, the anger coiled around me like a poisonous snake before I spat it out over others. As I grew into womanhood, the anger was still there—and I spat it out over my patients and bewildered husband, instead.

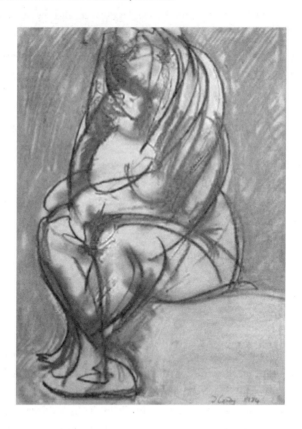

This "ice-cream" cone is my premenstrual self as painted by my sister, Zangmo (*www.creativewayart.com*), many moons ago. Zangmo is an artist, creativity coach, and Buddhist nun in the Tibetan tradition. For me, the picture encapsulates my energetic pain at the time.

Since those days my understanding and experience of my menstrual cycle has clarified, and the internal and external pain linked to my menstruation has eased for me now. I have come to terms with my feminine side and am aware that I can choose to handle my emotional, mental, and spiritual turbulence appropriately throughout the month, and not let it fester until a week before my bleed. Now, as a wise woman of menopausal energy, I work with younger women who wish to expand beyond their menstrual limitations and celebrate their spiritual connections.

My interest in the philosophy of the Wise Woman Tradition spans many years. For me, the weave of ancient eclectic beliefs and values combined with practical application and modern psychology has provided a natural pathway through the milestones of life. In this book, I would like to share with you some of the tools I use with both menstruating women and myself, and which you may like to work with on your special journey through your menstrual years. Choose instinctively, and travel with Spirit.

— Laurel

CHAPTER 1

Moving Through
the Menstrual Cycle

We begin to menstruate between 10 and 14 years old and continue until we reach 45–55 years of age. At that point, the natural menopausal transition heralds the cessation of monthly menstrual cycles and our child-bearing years.

Most women have menstrual cycles of about 28 days, but cycles can range from 21—36 days. A woman can be healthy and normal and have only a few cycles a year. If you have concerns, consult your GP or healthcare professional, as there may be an underlying condition affecting your menstrual cycle.

Did you know?

- You lose around 2 ounces of blood during a normal period (I sometimes feel like I lose a bucketful!).
- The length of your menstrual cycle (the number of days from the first day of your bleed to the first day of the next) is determined by the number of days it takes your ovary to release an egg. Once an egg is released, it normally takes about 14 days until menstruation occurs.
- When you are born, you have all the eggs your body will ever use—1–2 million eggs—but only a fraction of these will be released during your lifetime. When you start your periods, only about 300,000 eggs (stored in your ovaries) are still viable. As you mature into puberty, your body begins producing hormones that cause the eggs to mature.

This is the beginning of your first cycle, which will repeat throughout your life until the end of menopause and the cessations of monthly periods.

Menstrual Cycle

Follicular phase

The first phase is the follicular phase and begins on day 1 of your bleed, when the reproductive hormones estrogen and progesterone are at their lowest. The most active hormone at this stage is estradiol, the most potent of the three types of estrogen in the body. If fertilization doesn't occur, the spiral arteries of the lining close off, stopping blood flow to the surface of the lining. The blood pools into "venous lakes" that burst once they are full, and with the endometrial lining form your menstrual flow. Uterine cramping is one of the most common uncomfortable sensations women may have during menstruation. There are two kinds of cramping:

- **SPASMODIC CRAMPING:** Resulting from the production of prostaglandins, the hormone-like substances that regulate pain and inflammation in the body by causing either relaxation or constriction of the smooth muscles.
- **CONGESTIVE CRAMPING:** Resulting from possible food allergies (mainly wheat, dairy, or alcohol), which can increase estrogen levels, creating pelvic congestion and causing the body to retain fluids and salt.

The amount of blood that comes out of your vagina can be light, moderate, or heavy. The periods of some women start out light on the first day and then become heavy for a couple of days before lightening up. Others experience a light flow throughout their bleed. Still others have a heavy bleed all the way through. The length of the period varies from 2–7 days.

Towards the end of the bleed, there is likely to be an increase in energy and mood. Sleep patterns return to normal, appetite is regulated, and vaginal mucus is absent or dry. The follicular phase lasts 10–14 days, or until ovulation occurs.

Luteal phase

The second phase of your menstrual cycle is called the luteal phase. It begins when ovulation occurs. Ovulation is a process that begins when the level of luteinizing hormone surges, and ends 16–32 hours later with the release of an egg from one of your ovaries. Just before ovulation, your cervix secretes clear, slippery mucus, which helps facilitate the sperm's movement toward the egg. Inside the fallopian tube, the egg is carried along toward the uterus. As ovulation approaches, the blood supply to the ovary increases and the ligaments contract, pulling the ovary closer to the fallopian tube, allowing the released egg to find its way into the tube. Fertilization occurs if sperm are present. You may experience cramping (in the UK sometimes called *mittelschmerz,* a German word meaning "middle pain") in the area of either ovary. Ovulation pain may be caused by an emerging or ruptured follicle. A medical condition such as endometriosis, chronic pelvic inflammatory disease, or ovarian cyst could also be responsible. If you have regular ovulation pain, speak to your GP.

The luteal phase continues until day 1 of your next period. Your levels of estrogen and progesterone rise during this phase. These hormones work together to cause changes to the endometrial lining, preparing it for conception. If conception does not occur, levels of estrogen and progesterone decrease, causing the uterine lining to shed through menstruation. Towards the end of this phase, mucus may become drier and thicker as you enter the premenstrual time before you bleed.

WISE WOMAN WAYS

Here is a journey through your month from a sexual perspective:

DAY 1–7: Period starts. Your orgasmic potential is high due to increased testosterone.

DAY 8–14: Your rampant time, with testosterone peaking around day 14. This is when your body will get ready to release another egg, so it is also your most fertile time. A number of studies have suggested that a woman's vision and sense of smell are heightened at ovulation. Estrogen levels are starting to rise as your body gets ready for conception opportunities. Testosterone works to boost libido and energy, ensuring that the nipples and clitoris are sensitive to sexual arousal.

DAY 15–21: In the week following ovulation, progesterone levels increase and testosterone decreases, reducing sex drive.

DAY 21–28: Estrogen levels are low as your period approaches, which means you will have less natural lubrication. Testosterone lowers. Progesterone levels will have taken over.

Problems with periods

You may experience any of the following problems with your periods including:

- **AMENORRHEA:** This is the absence of a period in young women who haven't started menstruating by age 15 and women who haven't had a period for 90 days. Causes can include stress, breastfeeding, excessive exercising, severe weight loss, eating disorders, or serious medical conditions. Not having menstrual periods may mean that your ovaries have stopped producing normal amounts of estrogen. Hormonal issues, such as those caused by polycystic ovary syndrome (PCOS) may be involved. *Solution:* Talk to your GP or healthcare professional.

- **DYSMENORRHEA:** This describes painful period cramps. Menstrual cramps in teens are usually caused by excess prostaglandins. Period pain tends to happen when the muscular wall of the womb contracts, compressing the blood vessels that line your womb and temporarily cutting off the blood and oxygen supply to your womb. Without oxygen, the tissues in your womb release chemicals that trigger pain in your body. Occasionally, period pain can be caused by an underlying medical condition, such as fibroids, pelvic inflammatory disease, or endometriosis. Some cramping during the period is normal, due to the release of the hormone oxytocin (the hormone that causes contraction during birthing). *Solutions:* Massage, exercise, transcutaneous electronic nerve stimulation (TENS), hot water bottle, relaxation techniques, or a warm bath.

- **ABNORMAL UTERINE BLEEDING:** This term refers to vaginal bleeding that's different from normal menstrual periods. It includes bleeding or spotting between periods, bleeding after sex, and bleeding heavier or for more days than normal. Abnormal bleeding can have many causes. *Solution:* Talk to your GP or healthcare professional.

> **MENSTRUFACT**
> The same chemicals that cause uterine contractions during menstruation also cause the lower intestine to contract as well, which can lead to diarrhea.

What Happens Next?

Now we have an understanding of the how the menstrual cycle medically works, let's move on to a better understanding of the premenstrual syndrome in the next chapter.

CHAPTER 2

Premenstrual Syndrome

Premenstrual syndrome (PMS) describes a constellation of symptoms related to your menstrual cycle. Medical definitions of PMS refer to a pattern of emotional and physical symptoms that occur 5–10 days before menstruation that may interfere with some aspects of life and disappear shortly before or after the start of menstrual flow. There are four categories of PMS, according to renowned UK obstetrician, gynecologist, and endocrinologist Dr. Guy Abraham:

Type A - Anxiety

This category includes symptoms such as mood swings, irritability, anxiety, and nervous tension. Periods may start suddenly and be heavy with clots. Estrogen levels are high and progesterone levels low, which could be related to congestion in the liver and excess milk and animal fats.

Type C - Cravings

This category is associated with fluctuations in glucose levels in the body. Low blood sugar (hypoglycemia) and low levels of prostaglandins can cause headaches, fatigue, moodiness, and irritability and lead to increased appetite and food cravings, especially for sugar and chocolate. Other symptoms include dizziness, fainting, and heart palpitations.

Type H - Hyperhydration

With this category, water balance symptoms will occur, such as abdominal bloating, fluid retention, weight gain, bloating, breast tenderness and enlargement, and swollen hands and feet. These are related to high sodium and alcohol intake, possibly caused by elevated levels of the hormone aldosterone.

Type D – Depression

Changes such as depression, withdrawal, forgetfulness, clumsiness, lack of coordination, insomnia, confusion, and tearfulness are likely due to low estrogen and high progesterone levels. Magnesium levels seem to be low in this type. Heavy metal toxicity from lead may be another factor.

> **WISE WOMAN WAYS**
>
> In her book, *Energy Medicine*, Donna Eden makes a reference to PMS as a gift. PMS drops you deep into your own being, she suggests, and whatever you have been successful at burying or denying to yourself bursts forth at this time of the month. Personally, I have found this to be bang on. I listen carefully to my rants and raves at this time to discern any truths in them. Some of my rants are just hormone babble, while other raves contain kernels of truths and are worth listening to and maybe acting upon.

Constantly thinking about how bad your PMS symptoms are without taking positive action is not constructive. You are not helpless. You have a choice over how you handle your PMS. If you don't feel informed enough, become informed. If you need practical support, ask for it from friends or family. If you need conventional or complementary medical intervention, seek it.

During the run-up to your bleed, it isn't helpful to take out any negative feelings on yourself or others. Unleashing your anger on your nearest and dearest won't exactly enhance the relationship, and being constantly anxious can be counterproductive. So while yelling at someone or being in victim mode may feel justified in the moment, it may ultimately alienate someone close, achieve nothing, and make you feel guilty.

Some women are bothered by their PMS symptoms but don't deal with them directly; instead, they turn to expensive, self-destructive, or unhealthy behaviors to distract themselves, such as alcohol, drugs, isolation, shopping, or overeating. In the long run, it is better for your well-being (and for your bank balance and relationships) to manage your PMS symptoms like an adult, not a child.

Anti-inflammatories, diuretics, painkillers, and other medications can be helpful; ultimately, though, they may not be treating the causes of your PMS. The speed and efficiency of these drugs make it tempting to take a pill instead of making the adjustment towards a healthier lifestyle. I have to confess to doing this myself with painkillers, until I decided to work on my mindset. I asked myself what my pain was really about and how I learned to expect pain. Like many answers, mine lay in my past conditioning. When I made some psychological connections, my physical pain lessened. Then I learnt how to deal with the discomfort that was left through pain management. I still do take the occasional painkiller, especially if I am teaching a course. It's hard to focus in a mindful way on pain management when there is a sea of faces gazing at you for pearls of wisdom. Painkillers do the job then!

WISE WOMAN WAYS

Your body responds to how you think and feel. On a mind-body level, PMS may represent the resentment you may feel about having a period, feelings of being out of control, or conflicting emotions about femininity.

Understanding the mind-body connection in PMS is important because it will help you understand if there is something besides PMS at work. For example, if something in your lifestyle or personal situation is stressful, such as work, relationship issues, or financial problems, these could be exacerbating your symptoms. In order to ease the PMS, you may need to relieve the source of stress.

PMS may also worsen a number of medical conditions, including allergies, asthma, epilepsy, diabetes, multiple sclerosis (MS), lupus, and inflammatory bowel disease (IBS), and vice versa.

The estrogen and progesterone relationship affects PMS and can produce conditions such as fibroids and endometriosis. It may also have an influence on fertility, miscarriage, and premature birthing. Pregnancy complications, such as toxemia and pre-eclampsia, tend to occur when the woman has previously suffered from PMS.

Another thought is that the symptoms you attribute to PMS may actually be caused by another disease. If you are concerned about any PMS "symptom," consult your GP or healthcare professional, otherwise you could be jeopardizing your health.

Natural Remedies and Lifestyle Changes for PMS

Supplements *(see Chapter 4)*

- **CALCIUM** levels tend to be lower in the bodies of women with PMS, and supplementation can help reduce bloating, depression, pain, mood swings, and food cravings.
  NOTE: Calcium supplements should always be taken in combination with magnesium (see below), never alone.

Discuss with your GP before taking supplements, as recent scientific research suggests that calcium-only supplements may lead to a substantial increase in heart problems in those taking them, due to buildup of plaque in the body.

- **MAGNESIUM** is essential to the smooth functioning of the nervous system and is often chronically deficient in modern populations, due to its depletion in the soils in which our food is grown and demanding lifestyles. It calms the nervous system and improves mood, helps prevent weight gain, improves blood sugar balance, and can help reduce swelling of the hands and legs, breast tenderness, and abdominal bloating. NOTE: If you have heart or kidney disease, consult your GP before taking magnesium. Since mineral supplements may interact with antibiotics, blood pressure medications, diabetes medications, digoxin, the thyroid replacement medication levothyroxine, and osteoporosis medication, it's best if magnesium is only taken under medical supervision if you are managing any of those conditions.
- **VITAMIN B6** can taken for 10–14 days before your period or if you have general stress symptoms.
- **CHROMIUM GTF** may be taken for added help with cravings for sweet foods and general blood sugar imbalance.
- **HEMP SEED OIL** has a good balance of all three essential fatty acids (EFAs)—omegas 3, 6, and 9—which support brain balance. It has been shown to increase GLA levels in the body significantly, thereby easing PMS.
- **LINSEED (FLAXSEED) OIL** is good for very dry skin or eczema.
- **VITAMIN E** is indicated where there is breast tenderness.

Herbs *(see Chapter 5)*

- **VITEX AGNUS CASTUS** can reduce PMS symptoms such as irritability, depression, headaches, and breast tenderness by improving progesterone levels in the body. Take the tincture for three months from the middle of your cycle (ovulation) until you begin to menstruate. For best results take in the morning before rising for four cycles. **NOTE:** Vitex agnus castus may interact with hormones or drugs that affect the pituitary gland. If you suffer from pain around the time of ovulation, or you have a family history of ovarian cysts, consult a medical herbalist.
- **DANDELION LEAF** (either in capsule or tea form) encourages the elimination of excess water, while maintaining potassium levels.
- **RED CLOVER** tea can help to lower the effect of excess estrogen in the system.
- **EVENING PRIMROSE OIL** is an omega-6 EFA involved in the metabolism of prostaglandins, which regulate pain and inflammation in the body. It can be helpful for breast tenderness and needs to be taken for about three months to be effective. NOTE: EPO will not work as well if you regularly eat offal.
- **LICORICE** taken as a tea in the second half of the cycle is said to reduce estrogen and increase progesterone levels in the body. It also nourishes the adrenal glands, which are involved in the stress response and can become depleted when stress is prolonged. NOTE: Do not take licorice if you have high blood pressure or suffer from severe water retention. It can be very helpful for those with low blood pressure.

GENERAL NOTE: Avoid hormone-balancing herbs if you are on prescription hormonal medications such as the birth-control pill, synthetic (not bioidentical or natural) combination hormone replacement therapy (HRT) tablets, or tamoxifen.

> **WISE WOMAN WAYS**
>
> A lot of the anger and irritation women unleash during PMS is caused by poor communication skills. If you haven't learned to communicate well and tend to keep things bottled up, when your hormones fluctuate and your mood varies right before your period it is a prime opportunity to lash out. Learning to be an effective communicator will help you confront your problems as they occur—assertively as opposed to aggressively.

Progesterone cream *(see Chapter 4)*

Dietary recommendations *(see Chapter 4)*

Reduce the following:

- Table salt aggravates water retention and leads to bloating. Use unrefined sea salt instead, as it contains helpful minerals.
- Saturated fats, particularly from cheap supermarket meat, dairy, and eggs, and low-quality vegetable oils used in processed and refined foods such as store-bought cookies, cakes, and prepared frozen meals.
- Hydrogenated fats found in manufactured margarine and other processed foods.
- Refined sugar (including fructose and artificial sweeteners). Use small amounts of natural raw sweeteners, such as honey, maple syrup, and brown rice syrup instead.
- Caffeine.
- Alcohol. If you do drink, alternate each alcoholic drink with a glass of water. Limiting alcohol allows your liver to

function more effectively; the liver is responsible for detoxing the body, including clearing excess hormones (which cause hormonal imbalance) from the bloodstream. Alcohol consumption also contributes to blood sugar imbalance, which is implicated in PMS.

- Simple carbohydrates found in sweets and refined foods.

Increase the following:

- Foods that are high in complex carbohydrates, such as fresh fruits, vegetables, and whole grains. In particular, vegetables from the cabbage family (cruciferous vegetables) can increase the rate at which the liver changes estrogen into a water soluble form that can then be easily excreted. The cabbage family includes all cabbages, broccoli, Brussels sprouts, and radicchio.
- Organic foods, as they contain fewer hormones to interfere with the already turbulent confusion of hormones in your body.
- Grassfed meat, dairy, and eggs, as they contain high levels of vitamin D and omega 3 fats from the grass the animals eat, which improves well-being.
- Wild-caught salmon graze on algae, a mineral-rich and easily absorbable protein substance (such as spirulina or chlorella), which helps to correct blood sugar and anemia.
- Foods rich in calcium, in the form of milk and other dairy products, such as plain yogurt and cottage cheese. Vegan sources of absorbable calcium can be found in broccoli and beans.
- Legumes, including soybeans, chickpeas, lentils, mung beans, and aduki beans, contain important plant-based estrogens known as phytoestrogens, which help balance the

hormonal system, as do seeds, grains, and some herbs.

- Foods rich in omega 3 fatty acids, such as wild salmon and other oily fish, ground linseed, raw nuts, pumpkin seeds, hemp seeds, and fresh cold-pressed oils like extra virgin olive oil and linseed (flaxseed). To ensure adequate intake of omega 3 essential fatty acids, take a fish oil supplement. Although it is an incomplete omega 3 source, you can also use ground linseed (flaxseed) or its oil sprinkled on vegetables and salads, in smoothies, or taken by the spoonful.
- Water.

Exercise

Regular aerobic exercise, such as brisk walking, jogging, swimming, or cycling, may help relieve PMS symptoms. Personally speaking, if I get an urge to exercise, I lie down until it passes. I prefer lifestyle activities such as walking, gardening, or dancing.

Relaxation *(see Chapter 7)*

Breathing exercises, progressive muscular relaxation, meditation, aromatherapy, and yoga are some natural ways to reduce stress and promote relaxation.

Useful bodywork therapies

Chiropractic, massage, reflexology, or acupuncture may help relax you as well as relieve some of the symptoms of PMS.

Sleep

Many women have sleep problems during PMS. Inadequate sleep can impair your short-term memory, your judgment, your ability to process information, and your reaction times. You can improve sleep by practicing good sleep hygiene. Eliminate distractions in your bedroom (other than a lover!), including smartphones, computers, and TVs, which in addition to being distracting emit electromagnetic fields (EMFs) that affect the body. In addition, keep the room dark and the temperature cool to promote sleep. Lastly, avoid drinking caffeine and alcohol in the evening and before bedtime. Both are stimulants. If you still can't get a good night's rest during PMS, consider taking quick power naps that last only 20 minutes or so (ensure the nap is five hours away from bedtime).

Developing a positive mindset

If you look at PMS as a hopeless issue, you are thinking like a victim and will do very little to help yourself. Faulty thinking, where you generalize that everything is wrong because one thing hasn't gone as planned, is common with PMS. This pattern fuels your sense of helplessness and anger or anxiety. You need to recognize the faulty thoughts and replace them with positive mindsets and proactive behaviors. Knowing what causes PMS, learning what to expect each month, and finding ways to treat your symptoms are the best ways to manage PMS and prepare yourself both physically and psychologically for the experience. Take responsibility for your health, your habits, and your behaviors. It's one thing to acknowledge you have PMS; it's another thing to blame your negative behaviors on your condition. If you take responsibility, you will be more motivated to learn healthy new habits and find complementary or conventional healthcare solutions. Approaching PMS as a condition that you can easily treat will give you the mindset and ability to improve your situation.

WISE WOMAN WAYS

Teach your family and friends about PMS and how they can help you. For example, explain what they can do to help practically, when to leave you alone, or when a fresh perspective might ease the tension. Research has shown that strong social support systems, including closeness and connectedness, direct communication, and problem-solving skills, are inextricably linked to overall health and wellness.

MENSTRUFACT

Menstrual blood was thought to cure warts, birthmarks, gout, goiters, hemorrhoids, epilepsy, worms, leprosy, and headaches. The first sanitary napkin worn by a virgin was thought to be a cure for the plague. Menstrual blood was also used in love charms, to ward off demons, and was occasionally used as an offering to a god.

What Happens Next?

Understanding the menstrual cycle and gaining an eclectic awareness of PMS is only part of the story. Let us now explore the more spiritual aspects of menstruation.

CHAPTER 3

Cultural and
Spiritual Perspectives

According to C. Crawford[1], ancient people honored women for their apparently harmless monthly bleed and believed their ability to carry life within themselves as miraculous. Many centuries ago, menstruating woman were considered blessed (the word "blessing" derives from the Old English word, *bletsian,* meaning "bleeding"[2]).

Different Cultures
and Menstruation

Certain Native American cultures consider a menstruating woman to be at the height of her powers. For example, the Lakota tribe will not permit a menstrual woman near healers or warriors, as they believe that menstrual blood is so powerful it may weaken warrior strength and interfere with a healer's ability to heal. They believe menstrual blood serves to purify, cleanse, and renew a woman as she prepares for higher spiritual accomplishments. The tribe practices monthly rituals, whereby menstruating women retreat into "moon lodges" to celebrate the power of their menstrual blood.

Indians of South America believed that all humans were made of "moon blood" in the beginning. The Greeks believed the wisdom of man or god was centered in his blood, which came from his mother. Among the Ashanti, girl children are more prized than boys because a girl is the carrier of the blood. Chinese sages called menstrual blood the essence of Mother Earth, the yin principle, giving life to all things. A born-again ceremony from Australia showed the Aborigines linked rebirth with blood of the womb. Taoists believe that the menstrual flow is a primary contributor of qi for the female.

The Taoists, as well as the Celts, Persians, and Egyptians, practiced rituals where menstrual blood mixed with wine was considered sacred and powerful. For centuries before the appearance of Jesus Christ, red wine was a symbol of the Holy Woman or Great Mother. According to scholar Lawrence Durdin-Robertson[3], the name Charis (a goddess) means "grace" and is derived from the word for menstrual blood, which became the root for Eucharist. Red wine is now seen as a symbol of the blood of Christ, according to the Christian sacrament of communion.

> **WISE WOMAN WAYS**
>
> In ancient cultures women were the original shamans, and their spiritual beliefs were linked to the moon by both mental and blood cord. Female shamanism is based in the blood cycle (or blood mysteries) of birthing and menstruation. Just before and during menstruation, the female shaman experiences her strongest healing and oracular powers. On a physiological level, this makes sense: as estrogen levels rise in a woman's body, the levels of key neurotransmitters also rise, increasing the amount of adrenaline available for powerful healing.

In Ancient Greece spring festivals included the spreading on the earth of corn mixed with menstrual blood to increase fertility. Hindus in India tend to view first menstruation as a positive aspect of a girl's life. In South India, girls who experience their first period are given presents and celebrations to mark this special occasion. The Khoisan women of the Kalahari are considered most powerful when menstruating, and the "New Maiden" is given a special hut at this time.

> **WISE WOMAN WAYS**
> Wiccan and author Diane Stein's research shows that the original wand of power, rulership, and magick was the menstrual/birth/lunar calendar stick.

Hunter-Gatherer Societies

Until about 8,000 BC, our ancestors organized themselves into hunter-gatherer societies[4], with primitive religious beliefs that revolved around their nomadic, land-based lifestyle. Hunting was pivotal to tribal survival, and as a result, the hunter element in society (mostly men) tended to worship hunting gods and animals, such as the God of the Hunt or the Stag Horned God (or buffalo).

Women were mostly the gatherer element in society. They took care of the tribe and were the child bearers and healers. The female life-giving principle was considered divine, and the importance of fertility and birthing in crops, animals, and in the tribe itself was crucial to survival. As a result, women in hunter-gatherer societies tended to worship vegetative goddesses. While men and women might have worshipped similar gods and goddesses within the tribal community, they may also have gravitated to gender-specific worship. Women experienced a connection between their bodies and the phases of the moon that further enhanced the mystical link with the moon and the goddess deity. Because of these links, women during this time tended to lead the spiritual rituals of the tribe.

As society evolved, people began to settle in one place, growing food and breeding animals. This was when they became paganized (the word "pagan" is derived from the Latin word *paganus,* meaning "country dweller"). Paganism originates from the Neolithic (Stone Age) era. It was thought that everything had a spirit, so people had gods and goddesses for all aspects of their lives, including nature. Civilizations developed, and the gods were adapted to the changing lives of the people to play an important role in every aspect of the community.

The Triple Goddess

Long before the advent of Christianity, the Temple in Jerusalem had a tower representing the Great Goddess in her triple aspect. Known as Mari (a possible ancient Goddess source influencing the later worship of Mary and the Virgin Mother), the images shown are the three stages of the female life cycle: the premenstrual maiden, the fertile menstrual nymph, and the postmenopausal crone[5].

The term "neopagan"[6] encompasses a broad definition used for a wide variety of modern religious or spiritual concepts influenced by the pre-Christian pagan beliefs of Europe. Wicca (popularly called White Witchcraft, the benign religion of the ancient Celts and an example of neopaganism) reemerged in the mid-20th century in England. Not only does Wicca tend to honor the Triple Goddess of maiden (virginity), mother (fertility), and crone (wisdom)[7], but it also honors the Horned God. These two deities are often viewed as being a sacred blend of nature (or the universe) and the Divine. The Maid-Mother-Crone symbolizes the following phases:

- The Maid of childhood and adolescence: youth and possibility, emerging sexuality;
- The Mother of child-bearing years: creativity and nurturing; and
- The Crone of the menopausal years: wisdom transition, the compassion that comes from experience, and the one who guides us through the death and rebirth experience.

Each phase of the Triple Goddess represents a different type of healing and growth in a woman's life. Her aspects are mirrored in the phases of the moon: new, waxing, full, and waning. This goddess philosophy linking spirituality and earth cycles can be found across many time frames and cultures, including Norse, Greek, Hindu, Celtic, and Roman belief systems.

The goddess and menstruation

Indigenous peoples understood the power inherent in menstrual blood, which in particular was seen to embody the creative energy of the Goddess.

The Hindu Kuala Tantra sees a menstruating woman as the living embodiment of the Goddess Kali. Her menstrual blood is the life essence of humankind and all creation, a potent rejuvenating and transforming force. Egyptian pharaohs became divine by ingesting *sa,* the blood of the Goddess Isis. The hieroglyphic sign for sa was the same as the sign for the vulva: a symbol similar to a yonic loop such as the ankh, or Cross of Life. Chinese sages called menstrual blood the essence of Mother Earth, the yin principle, giving life to all things.

In Mesopotamia, the Great Goddess created people out of clay and infused them with her blood of life. She taught women to form clay dolls and to smear them with menstrual blood. The name Adam translates as "bloody clay." In Hindu theory, as the Great Mother created the earth, solid matter coalesced into a clot with a crust. Women use this same method to produce new life.

> **WISE WOMAN WAYS**
>
> *A TRADITIONAL MOON CYCLE*
>
> Your monthly bleed has finished, and you are now in the Maiden aspect of your Goddess energy. At this time, you are energetically reborn and able to expand and direct your attention to the outside world.

This, for many women, is the time of the new moon, when you are mentally focused, rational, and practical. Celebrate this time as one where you can synthesize new ideas into a workable whole. As your estrogen rises, this is an easy time to feel courageous and tireless, using your intelligence to improve your life.

For many of you, this phase is halfway through your cycle (some of you may bleed on the full moon and not on the new moon). Now you are in the Mother aspect of your Goddess energy, the time of full moon and ovulation. You are the giver of life and abundance, ripe, full of love and passion. It is a time to value relationship, partnership, and the well-being of others. Your satisfaction comes from engaging with the supporting, receptive, and nurturing roles of your life partially due to progesterone, the mothering hormone.

You are now in the time after ovulation and before menstruation. The Enchantress phase of your Goddess energy is when you may experience dissatisfaction about particular aspects of your life. This is the time to be meditative and spiritually orientated. Spend some time alone, working creatively to hear the messages from within. This phase prepares you for the release and letting go as you enter the (Crone) bleeding phase of your cycle.

The premenstrual time is a phase of the waning moon (as the moon goes from full to dark), when your energy turns inward and your intuition is at its height. Now you are in the Crone aspect of your Goddess energy, which relates to the bleeding phase in the menstrual cycle. The Crone is the one who dissolves and takes away that which is no longer needed.

> This is the time when you can focus on yourself rather than constantly nurturing others. The Crone sees the truth everywhere in your life, relationships, and actions and She will work upon you to clear out that which you no longer need.

Cross-Cultural Words and Expressions for Menstruation

All cultures across the world have idiomatic expressions for menstruation. With thanks to the Museum of Menstruation & Women's Health, Maryland, United States[8], here are some for your interest:

- "Having visitors" (Zambia)
- *Mae hi yn ei bodau* meaning "she is in her flowers" (Wales)
- Fairy hammocks (England). (British comedienne Jo Brand once referred to sanitary towels as "Fairy Hammocks")
- *El inquilino comunista* meaning "the communist guest" (Spain)
- *Rooi gety* meaning "red tide" (South Africa, Afrikaans language)
- "Old faithful" (America)
- *Imam zenske muke* meaning "I have female trouble" (Serbia)
- "Bleeding like a banshee" (Scotland)
- *Techka* meaning "drippage" or "flow" (Russia)
- *¿Te canto el gallo?* meaning "did the rooster already sing?" (Puerto Rico)
- *Estou com a fita vermelha na máquina* meaning "I have the red label in the old typewriter" (Portugal)
- *Ciocia z Moskwy* meaning "Aunt from Moscow" (Poland)
- "Up on blocks" (Northern Ireland)

- "Doing time" (Nigeria)
- "Red sails in the sunset" (New Zealand)
- *De dam van de Rode Zee is gebroken* meaning "the dam from the Red Sea has broken" (The Netherlands)
- "I'm having my lady's period" (Jamaica)
- "Liverpool's playing at home" (Ireland). *(Comment from Laurel: My husband is an Arsenal fan—needless to say there is an English equivalent for this Irish expression: Arsenal are playing at home)*
- "The red snow" (India)
- "Mother's eldest sister" (China). Pads are called "mother's eldest sister napkins" in China.
- "Bitchy-witchy week" (America)

MENSTRUFACT
Tampon is French for "plug" or "bung," a variant from the Old French word *tapon*, meaning a "piece of cloth to stop a hole." Before the creation of tampons in the 1920s, Western women used washable and reusable rags.

What Happens Next?

We can see that the journey through the menstrual cycle can be full of inner symbolism. Working with this can help us to make some sense of our spiritual and psychological journey. However, we mustn't forget to nourish our physical body through good nutrition. The next chapter sets out recommended supplements and foods for a range of menstrual symptoms.

CHAPTER 4

Good Nutrition

In addition to providing a healthy mind and body, good food supplies the raw materials your neuroendocrine (nerve-hormone) system needs to create healthy hormonal and emotional balance as you go through your monthly cycle.

> **WISE WOMAN WAYS**
>
> The most common craving during the menstrual cycle is for chocolate, which can be an indication of magnesium deficiency. A magnesium supplement? Or chocolate? I think I'll go for the 70 percent cocoa supplement!

Progesterone and Menstruation

Progesterone is the hormone produced by the female ovaries after ovulation. It supports and maintains pregnancy, is the precursor to other vital hormones, and is needed to balance estrogen levels. Estrogen promotes cell growth, and progesterone keeps that growth from going farther than is healthy. Your estrogen levels may be unbalanced if your body is not producing enough progesterone.

Most women begin to produce less progesterone in their early 30s, and this loss accelerates in their 40s. This progesterone deficiency can cause perimenopause symptoms.

The use of bioidentical or natural progesterone cream to treat female hormonal issues was pioneered by the late Dr. John Lee,[9] a Californian family doctor. It is made in the laboratory from plant sources such as Mexican yam and, as the term "bioidentical" indicates, it is identical to the hormone produced by the ovaries. Natural proges-terone can be used to help support menstrual issues, such as irregular menstrual flow, bloating, depression, irritability, insomnia, and low sex drive.

NOTE: Bioidentical or natural progesterone cream is readily available over the counter in a basic strength in health food stores like Whole Foods in the United States, as well as by specific-strength pre-scription from your doctor through special compounding pharmacies. The situation in the United Kingdom is different, however. Bioidenti-cal progesterone cream is not licensed for medical use in the United Kingdom, and as a result, is only available as an unlicensed medicine by prescription from your doctor. If you choose not to consult a doc-tor, you can legally import bioidentical progesterone cream from outside the United Kingdom, provided it is solely for your own use. Several well-known companies, such as Emerita (Progest), make their products available in the United Kingdom.[10]

Vitex agnus castus is said to work at the level of the pituitary gland and can increase progesterone production. Take it consistently for a few months in tincture form. Evening primrose may boost progester-one levels, although its main role is balancing both progesterone and estrogen and bringing them to their correct levels.

Phytoestrogen foods

Phytoestrogens are weak estrogen-like compounds in plants (*phyto* means plant). They lock onto and block estrogen receptors, making it harder for harmful chemicals to disrupt hormone signals. It is thought that phytonutrients act as hormone regulators, rather than mimicking estrogen or progesterone.

Food sources include oats, barley, rye, brown rice, couscous, bulgur wheat, sunflower seeds, sesame seeds, pumpkin seeds, poppy, linseeds (flaxseeds), tofu, whole soy products (except soy sauce), citrus, chickpeas, kidney beans, haricot beans, broad beans, green split peas, red onions, green beans, celery, sweet peppers, garlic, broccoli, tomatoes, rhubarb, apples, aniseed, brewers yeast, beetroot, cabbage, carrots, clover, corn, cucumbers, green squash, olives, olive oil, papaya, peas, plums, potatoes, legumes, nuts, squash, cherries, dried dates, hummus, alfalfa sprouts, dried apricots, and mung bean sprouts.

Foods to Include During
Your Monthly Cycle

Your daily meals should include a variety of foods from the four main food groups:

- **FRUITS AND VEGETABLES:** You can buy these fresh, frozen, dried, or juiced. Fresh or frozen are the best sources, as these methods retain the important nutrients. Aim for five servings a day.
- **CARBOHYDRATES:** These include starchy foods like bread, pasta, rice, and potatoes. Try to choose whole grains (complex carbohydrates), which digest more slowly, thereby keeping your energy even all day. Have around four servings of whole grains, such as bread, cereals, pasta, rice, noodles, yams, and potatoes, per day.
- **PROTEIN:** These include lean meat and chicken; pasteurized dairy products, such as milk, cheese, and yoghurt; fish; eggs; and pulses (such as beans and lentils). Try to aim for at least two portions of fish a week, particularly including wild-caught oily fish like wild salmon, halibut, and sardines, which are high in essential omega 3 fats and a natural source of vitamin D, the "sunshine" vitamin.
- **FATS:** Essential fatty acids are good fats that are essential to your health. Omega 3 fatty acids can ease the symptoms of PCOS, endometriosis, menstrual cramps, and PMS through their

anti-inflammatory properties. Good sources include grassfed meats, dairy, and egg products; wild game; coldwater fish, such as wild-caught Alaskan salmon and halibut; fermented soy products, such as tofu and miso; flax seeds; oily nuts, such as walnuts; unprocessed canola oil and cold-pressed extra-virgin olive oil; leafy green vegetables, such as spinach and kale; and cruciferous vegetables, such as broccoli, cauliflower, and cabbage. Note, too, that research has shown some important health benefits from real butter—that is organic pastured (grassfed) butter, as opposed to spreads and margarines. Butter is a natural food essential to your health, whereas margarine is a man-made food product made from refined polyunsaturated oils that are hydrogenated chemically and potentially more detrimental to health than saturated fat. Quality butter contains lecithin for cholesterol metabolism and antioxidants that protect against free radical damage, plus it is a great source of vitamins A, D, E, and K; omega 3s; conjugated linoleic acids (which has been shown to help prevent cancer); and the minerals selenium and iodine. I also recommend organic butter from grassfed cows because it lessens exposure to toxic substances such as pesticides that could be harmful to health.

Insomnia

Recommended supplements

- Calcium/magnesium
- Multivitamin/mineral
- Vitamin B complex
- GTF chromium (at lunchtime)
- 5HTP, a naturally occurring amino acid, a precursor to the neurotransmitter serotonin, and an intermediate in trypto-phan metabolism.

- Trytophan boosts serotonin, the feel-good neurotransmitter in the brain that is also used by the pineal gland to make melatonin, the hormone that controls the sleep/wake cycle. You could take a melatonin supplement, if you don't have any success with 5HTP, tryptophan foods, and so on, but be cautious and start with a very low level of the hormone; it does not agree with everyone. It must be taken in the early evening, several hours before bedtime, in order to work.

Best foods

- A common reason for insomnia is low blood sugar (hypo-glycemia), which is why some people wake in the middle of the night or early morning feeling hungry. If the blood glucose falls too low after eating too lightly or the wrong foods the evening before, and there are no glycogen stores in the muscles for the body to convert to glucose to get through the night, it is a potentially dangerous situation for the brain, which depends on glucose to control body processes. A drop in glucose levels promotes the release of glucose-regulating hormones (adrenalin, glucagon, cortisol, and growth hormone), and this wakes you up. For these people, it is important to eat food that is slow burning, such as oat cakes, cereal, whole-grain bread, a soft pretzel, bagels, or whole-grain crackers accompanied by a small amount of lean protein. Pomegranates are believed to induce sleep.
- Tryptophan is an amino acid that helps the brain produce serotonin, a natural sedative. It is found in bananas, peanuts, shrimps, cod, soybeans, braised calves liver, roast turkey, roasted chicken breast, boiled spinach, boiled as-paragus, kale, cauliflower, broccoli, boiled egg, and heated

goat's and cow's milk. Adding honey to warm milk helps
get the tryptophan in your system faster.

Any food allergy may cause poor sleeping and insomnia. Foods causing allergic reactions are known to increase heart rate among other
reactions, causing or aggravating insomnia. Food additives, colorings,
and preservatives should also be avoided.

Avoid stimulant drugs, painkillers containing caffeine, cigarettes,
and alcohol. Slimming tablets contain strong stimulants and make
it hard to sleep, as do street drugs like Ecstasy, cocaine, and amphet-
amines.

Avoid all refined carbohydrates, especially sugar, pastries, white
flour, white rice, and other processed foods, as they spike your blood
sugar and cause rapid highs and lows that stress the body. Excess use of
table salt has also been frequently associated with insomnia (although
unrefined sea salt, with its high level of minerals, can be very calming). Avoid caffeine, and don't eat a big meal or spicy foods just before
bedtime.

Fatigue

Recommended supplements

- Active coenzyme form of vitamin B3
- L-carnitine
- Potassium-magnesium aspartate
- Vitamin B12
- Asian ginseng
- Fish oil
- Licorice

Best foods

- Whole grains, organ meats, sweet potatoes, avocados, egg yolks, fish, and whey. Both oatstraw and nettle infusions are good sources of B vitamins.
- Vitamin C foods, such as cantaloupe, citrus fruit and juices, kiwi, pineapple, strawberries, raspberries, broccoli, Brussels sprouts, cauliflower, green and red peppers, spinach, and tomatoes. Cooking reduces the availability of vitamin C in food. Microwaving or steaming foods improve availability. The best food sources of vitamin C are raw fruits and vegetables.
- Tired women need more high-quality fuel, including good fats, in their diet, especially natural sources of vitamin E, such as avocados, peanut butter, sunflower seeds, tahini, and cold-pressed extra-virgin olive oil. Herbs rich in vitamin E include nettle, seaweeds, dandelion, and watercress.
- Celery, cabbage, seaweeds, nettle infusion, and red clover infusion are excellent sources of potassium.
- For iodine, consume seaweeds, unprocessed sea salt, mushrooms, and leafy greens grown in gardens fertilized with seaweed.
- You may need to increase your intake of iron. Consume a spoonful of blackstrap molasses or take a dropperful of yellow dock tincture several times a day. Good food sources include seaweeds, nettle infusion, dandelion leaves, cocoa powder and chocolate (yippee!), tahini, broccoli, spinach, sundried tomatoes, chicken, parsley, turkey, roasted pumpkin and squash seeds, sunflower seeds, kale, lentils, watercress, toasted sesame seeds, cooked egg yolks, apricots (fresh or dried), fish, red meat, and haricot beans.
- The following foods are naturally high in vitamins and minerals and will help you sustain energy throughout the day and are good late-evening snacks to help you sleep:

42

- Peanut butter and almond butter
- Live-culture yoghurt
- Slightly underripe banana
- Cheese and oatcakes
- Turkey breast sandwich
- Hard-boiled egg
- Chicken salad on whole-wheat pita bread
- Pasta salad
- Baked potato with low-fat cheese topping

I have found one of the best solutions for fatigue, apart from resting my body and mind, is to eat little and often. Breakfast is an oaty-based cereal, scrambled or poached egg on granary toast, or probiotic yoghurt with fruit. Lunch is normally a slice of Scandinavian crispbread, such as Ryvita, or granary bread with some protein and salad, followed by pineapple or licorice. Supper is fish or lean meat with salad or other vegetables. Snacks include fruit mid-morning and rye bread mid-afternoon.

Water Retention

Recommended supplements

- Selenium

Best foods

- Foods that relieve water retention include asparagus, nettles, corn (and corn silk tea), grapes, cucumbers, watermelon (and watermelon seed tea), parsley, celery, and black tea and green tea (no more than 2 cups a day).
- Avoid eating too much regular table salt. Use unrefined sea salt.

Constipation

Recommended supplements

- Garlic capsules
- Aloe vera juice
- Flaxseed oil

Best foods

- Add fiber to your diet through healthier snacks, such as fruit, popcorn, nuts, and vegetable sticks.
- Eat more servings of high-quality, lean red meat and dark-green vegetables, such as broccoli, kale, carrots, spinach, Brussels sprouts, asparagus, and green leafy cabbage.
- Start your day with a cup of warm water with a slice of lemon in it (great for the skin, too).
- Start each meal with salad or fruit, to increase your intake of high-fiber foods (roughage) and vitamin C.
- Eat fresh, dried, or frozen fruits, including oranges, grapefruits, dried prunes, apricots, apples, bananas, blackberries, figs, grapes, peaches, plums, raspberries, strawberries, figs, pears, papaya, and pineapple.
- Consume blackstrap molasses, if you need a good natural laxative. Take a tablespoonful last thing at night.
- Eat more fresh vegetables including celery, watercress, cabbage, spinach, and artichokes.
- Up your intake of whole-grain cereals and bread, beans, lentils, and other pulses that contain fiber.
- Psyllium or ispagula husks, the seeds from plantain, have been shown in some research to be effective for constipation, particularly in those with IBS.
- A glass of freshly made raw cabbage juice or juiced zucchini works well.

- I always recommend linseeds (flaxseeds), which are rich in fiber and essential fatty acids, for constipation. Keep the seeds in the freezer to keep their fats fresh and unspoiled, grind the seeds as you need them, and sprinkle on foods, in smoothies, yoghurt, even salads. Alternatively, you can buy high-quality, high-lignin linseed oil in a dark bottle (freezer sections of natural grocery stores) and either use it as a salad oil or eat by the teaspoon (a bit *urgh* in my experience, as un-refined linseed oil has a very strong taste and smell, a bit like turpentine. However, refined versions are now available that taste better, as well as versions that are flavored with lemon). NOTE: Be sure to keep all of these healthy vegetable oils in the fridge, as they spoil rapidly when exposed to air and particularly light (this is why they are usually in dark bottles). Buy small quantities and use them up fast to get maximum benefit.
- If you use bran to manage constipation, simultaneously increase your fluid intake, as without extra water, bran will make your stool hard and difficult to pass along the intestines.
- A can of sauerkraut, juice and all, is a fine laxative.
- A high-fiber diet provides more roughage to help digestion, but remember to increase your fluid intake to at least 1.5 liters (2.6 pints) of water daily.

Avoid drinks that are diuretics (make you pass more urine), such as black tea, coffee, cola and alcohol, as these can dehydrate you, making constipation worse. Drink plain filtered water, barley water, and cranberry juice.

WISE WOMAN WAYS

USING THE SQUAT FOR CONSTIPATION

The following may not be dinner party reading, but the information may help you manage your bowel movements better: change postures when you go to the loo. When you sit, your puborectalis muscle restricts the rectum in order to maintain "continence," thereby kinking it and sometimes resulting in unfinished or constrictive bowel movements. A relaxed, full squat posture (popular in yoga—Indians make good use of the squat position—and useful for birthing!) relaxes the puborectalis muscle, straightens the rectum, and facilitates complete bowel movements. Several websites sell products that make squatting to evacuate the bowels more comfortable, including *www.naturesplatform.com* or *www.toilet-related-ailments.com/index.html.*

Menstrual Flooding

A hormonal imbalance, linked to high estrogen, fluctuating progesterone, and a sluggish liver, is the most common cause of heavy menstrual bleeding. Uterine fibroid tumors are another common cause of excessive menstruation. Cervical polyps are small growths, the cause of which is not clear; however, they are often the result of an infection and many times associated with an abnormal response to increased estrogen levels or congestion of the blood vessels located in the cervix. Other causes of heavy menstruation include endometrial polyps, pelvic inflammatory disease (PID), and intrauterine devices (IUDs).

Recommended supplements

- Vitamin K deficiency can cause heavy menstrual periods. If you bleed heavily but don't see a lot of clotting and you

bruise easily, you could be suffering from vitamin K deficiency. It is best to get your vitamin K from foods rather than
supplements. You'll find it in leafy green vegetables such as
broccoli, cauliflower, spinach, and parsley.

- Vitamin E has been used to treat heavy periods. Avoid very
large amounts, as it can cause blood thinning.

- Essential fatty acids (EFAs) can be used to calm flooding.
Take capsules or tablespoons of flaxseed oil, borage seed
oil, blackcurrant seed oil, or evening primrose oil. Borage,
blackcurrant, and evening primrose oils are all high in GLA
(gamma linoleic acid).

- Iron

- Flavonoids

- Vitamin C

- Vitamin A

Best foods

- If you bleed heavily, you may need extra iron to replace the
iron that is being lost. Take iron in several small doses in the
day rather than one large dose. Acids and proteins (citrus
juice or dairy, for example) increase iron uptake in foods
that contain iron, such as spinach, so combine the two for
absorption by squeezing lemon juice on your greens or eating
them with yoghurt. You may also take a liquid iron supplement, such as Floradix, during periods of heavy bleeding.
Blackstrap molasses is an excellent source of iron. For better
absorption, don't drink black tea with iron supplements or
meals that contain iron. Coffee, soy foods, egg yolks, bran,
and calcium supplements of over 250mg impair iron absorption. NOTE: Do not take iron supplements unless you are
under medical supervision for anemia, as taking iron when

you don't need it is dangerous. Upping your food sources should not be a problem, though, and, in fact, is highly recommended.

- Supplement your diet with plenty of iron-rich, dark-green leafy vegetables and root vegetables, egg yolks, liver, red meat, raisins and prunes, high-quality protein, and whole grains.
- Reduce saturated animal fats, which are converted by the body into estrogens, thereby confusing feedback mechanisms. Organic, grass-fed, lean meats do not contain supplemental hormones or antibiotics and are best.
- Linseed (flaxseed) can be taken in the form of flaxseed oil or by grinding refrigerated flaxseeds as you need them and sprinkling on cereal, salad, or vegetables or as part of a smoothie. Consume linseed first thing in the morning, and drink a glass of water or herb infusion at the same time. Be sure to keep linseed or its oil refrigerated, to avoid the delicate oils turning rancid and causing inflammation in the body.

Avoid aspirin and specially formulated premenstrual pain relievers such as Midol, as they thin the blood (as does coumarin) and may increase bleeding. Also avoid blood-thinning herbs such as red clover, alfalfa, cleavers, pennyroyal, willow bark, and wintergreen. Thin blood is more likely to hemorrhage. Garlic can also thin the blood.

I began to take serious notice of my nutrition when I was diagnosed with breast cancer many moons ago. Have to confess, though—I'm a foodie! I eat healthy food for my bowels (constipation can be an issue if I'm stressed), to keep my bad (LDL) cholesterol in check (it's a tad high), and for my liver (you must keep the liver functioning well in order to get rid of excess hormones and toxins). I also use supplements such as bee propolis during the winter months. I occasionally fall off the good food wagon, happily have a ball, then get back to healthy eating. A little of what I fancy does me the world of good!

> **WISE WOMAN WAYS**
> Seaweeds of all kinds help restore energy by nourishing the body's vital nervous, immune, and endocrine systems. Make it a habit to eat seaweed as a green vegetable at least once a week. Try kelp in your oatmeal, wakame in your beans, kombu in your soups, hijiki salads, toasted dulse, sea palm fronds, and deep-fried nori and sushi.

Fibroids

Uterine fibroids occur frequently in up to half of all women over 40. They are growths of smooth muscle and fibrous tissue of widely varying size in the uterus, but they may become very large. The great majority of fibroids show no symptoms, but some may cause abnormal menstrual bleeding and symptoms of pressure on the bladder that may cause you to urinate frequently.

Fibroids occur during the reproductive years, when estrogen and progesterone levels are at their highest; after menopause they disappear, as estrogen levels that feed the fibroids steeply decline. But because estrogen levels can rise during the late perimenopausal years, due to estrogen dominance, previously asymptomatic fibroids may grow in the years just before the cessation of menses. This results in symptoms such as a feeling of heaviness in the belly, lower back pain, pain during vaginal penetration, urinary frequency or incontinence, bowel difficulties, or severe menstrual pain and flooding.

Where there is estrogen dominance in the body, progesterone balances out the excess. When enough progesterone is supplied, fibroid growth is arrested. Normally, the liver can easily deal with slight excesses of estrogen, but if your diet is poor, you suffer from allergies, or take in excess toxins, your liver's ability to detoxify and eliminate estrogen can be impaired (a herbal detox may be a good idea). Increase nutrients in the diet. Follow a hormone-balancing diet consisting of lots of fresh fruits and vegetables, adequate protein, complex carbohydrates such as whole grains, and moderate amounts of healthy fat. Counter excess estrogen with phytoestrogenic foods such as flaxseed and soy.

Recommended supplements

- Vitamin B complex
- Beta carotene
- Zinc picolinate or zinc citrate
- Vitamin E of d-alpha tocopherol
- Linseed (flaxseed) oil
- Vitamin C
- Apply topical bioidentical progesterone cream to counter the effects of overproduction of estrogen, otherwise known as estrogen dominance.

Best foods

- Eat organic fruit and vegetables.
- Filter your drinking water.
- Whole grains are full of lignins (compounds that have an antiestrogenic effect on the body). Eat plenty of rye, millet, whole soy (especially fermented soy products such as miso and tempeh and natto, fermented soybeans), oats, buckwheat, barley, corn, and brown rice.
- Consume two tablespoons of cracked linseed (flaxseed) each day. Sprinkle in smoothies, yoghurt, soups, salads, stir fries, or on baked potatoes.

- Reduce your intake of saturated animal fats. Healthy essential fats found in nuts and seeds are fine.
- A good guideline is to eat 50 percent of your foods in their raw state each day.
- Avoid coffee, cocoa, flour products, dairy, chocolate, and sugar, and stay away from cheap, junk fats, margarine, and poor-quality vegetable cooking oils.
- Make sure that vegetables are thoroughly washed with apple cider vinegar or lemon juice to help remove the pesticides, as these affect the body much like synthetic estrogen. Ideally, choose organic vegetables, which are untreated with pesticides.
- Make sure you eat a high-fiber diet.
- Limit meat to three times a week. Cheaply produced meat and dairy products from animals raised in crowded, unsanitary conditions on large feedlots contain significant amounts of antibiotics to keep the animals healthy and estrogen from being treated with hormones to speed up animal growth. High-quality proteins such as organic grassfed meat and dairy, free-range eggs, and wild-caught fish may cost a little more but they are an important investment in your health: you won't need to eat as much in order to feel satisfied, they contain no added hormones or antibiotics, and have been shown to have significantly higher levels of omega 3 essential fatty acids, vitamin D, conjugated linoleic acid (CLA), and other health-promoting nutrients. Vegetable protein sources contain beneficial complex carbohydrates and are less acid forming than meat.
- High-quality protein foods that have a good balance of amino acids include free-range eggs, quinoa (an ancient grain that cooks like rice), seed vegetables (runner beans, peas, corn, broccoli), cottage cheese, nuts and seeds, soy (tofu), organic meat and fish, and beans and lentils.

Decrease stress

When you take in a stimulant, such as coffee, or react stressfully to an event, the body produces the essential adrenal hormone cortisol. This hormone competes with progesterone for receptor sites (sites within the body that would normally receive progesterone to balance out the estrogen). As a result, the effect of being in an ongoing stressed state is less active progesterone in the body. Cortisol also increases production of estrogen, so prolonged stress can contribute to estrogen dominance.

Finally, lose excess body fat and do regular exercise, especially strength training.

> **WISE WOMAN WAYS**
>
> Fibroids, suggests wholistic physician Christiane Northrup[11], are symbolic of creativity waiting to be birthed and may also result when we are putting our life force into relationships (personal or professional) that have no meaning for us. Consider:
>
> - What creations within me do I wish to bring into existence?
> - If I could have or be anything, how would I choose to live my life?
> - If I had six months to live, who would I choose to be with for nourishment and inspiration?

An Important Note on Menstrual
Cramping and Vitamin D

Vitamin D is not actually a vitamin; it's an essential fat-soluble hormone made through skin exposure to the sun, hence its nickname: the "sunshine vitamin." Vitamin D is necessary for calcium absorption and absorbed as either cholecalciferol (vitamin D3) or ergocalciferol (vitamin D2). Deficiency can contribute to rickets and other bone problems, some cancers, and multiple sclerosis and would appear to influence the immune system. In many regions around the world, including the United States, vitamin D deficiency is common because people do not spend enough time in the sun to facilitate the hormone's production. The body also makes less vitamin D as you age—typically someone in their 70s makes 75 percent less vitamin D than someone in their 20s, leading to chronic vitamin D deficiency in the elderly.

Upping your vitamin D intake has been shown to help relieve some of the distress associated with menstrual cramping. That's because hormone-like substances called prostaglandins trigger the uterus to contract during menstruation as a means of expelling the uterine lining. These substances are associated with inflammation and pain, and high levels are linked to menstrual cramps. Vitamin D helps to decrease both the production of prostaglandins and cytokines, which promote inflammation in your body.

You cannot get adequate vitamin D through dietary sources alone, but upping your consumption of foods fortified with vitamin D, such as cereal flours and milk, and foods naturally containing vitamin D is very helpful. Alfalfa and mushrooms (shiitake and portabella) are good sources of vitamin D2. Free-range egg yolks, beef liver, and wild-caught fatty fishes such as eel, catfish, tuna, salmon, sardines, and mackerel are good sources of vitamin D3, the more important of the two D vitamins.

The ideal (and most pleasant) way to increase vitamin D levels is through safe sun exposure. Take a "sun bath" for 15–20 minutes a day (depending on where you live and the strength of the sun), which should net you 10,000 IU (international units) of vitamin D, a recommended daily dosage to top up vitamin D stores naturally for health. It's important to expose large areas of your skin to the sun as close to midday as possible in order to receive the correct UV rays for vitamin D production. Limit exposure to just the point when your skin starts to turn pink, then cover up and use your usual sunscreen for the rest of the day to protect the skin.

Realistically, it can be very hard to get adequate therapeutic vitamin D from sun exposure in northern latitudes with inadequate sunshine, such as Britain, and modern lifestyles increasingly mean that we are indoors much of the time, so you may well need to take a daily over-the-counter (OTC) oral vitamin D3 supplement for health. The suggested dosage will depend very much on where you live, your sun exposure, your age, your lifestyle, and the vitamn D levels in your body. It is true that many studies are indicating that very high dosages under medical supervision (300,000 IU in one study on menstrual cramping) have been shown to be effective in correcting deficiencies and health problems; however, it is theoretically possible to overdose on vitamin D when taken at extremely high doses in supplement form, especially when your vitamin A (not beta carotene) and vitamin K2 are not properly balanced. Megadoses may also lead to damaging deposits of calcium in your heart, lungs, or kidneys.

Currently, both the US and UK governments are very conservative in their general recommendations for vitamin D supplementation. In the United States, FDA guidelines for vitamin D are 600 IU daily for healthy people, but due to the chronic deficiencies now being found in the general population, many American doctors now recommend 4,000–10,000 IU, to maintain adequate vitamin D in the body. For this reason, it is essential to get your D3 levels tested, then work with your doctor to maintain therapeutic levels in the body (40–60 ng/ml). Remember: you cannot overdose on vitamin D from sun exposure—the way our bodies evolved to get large doses of vitamin D daily—and this is all the more reason to get adequate sun exposure on a daily basis.

MENSTRUFACT

According to Dr. Carol Livoti and Elizabeth Topp,[12] during prehistoric times, a woman had 50 menstrual cycles in her lifetime. Today, women in agricultural regions menstruate about 150 times in a lifetime, and the average woman in a modern industrialized society menstruates 450 times in her life.

What Happens Next?

A nourishing diet during our monthly cycle will help our bodies deal with the changing hormones. As Wise Women, we also know the value of using herbs as part of our daily nutrition. I cover this in the chapter that follows.

Useful Resources

Organizations

- British Association for Applied Nutrition and Nutritional Therapy, *www.bant.org.uk* (for listings of qualified nutritional therapists)
- American Dietetic Association, *www.eatright.org* (for registered dietitians)

Supplements

The Nutri Centre, *www.nutricentre.com*

CHAPTER 5

Wort Cunning

The Wise Woman going through her menstruation years will embrace the use of herbs (ideally organic) into her healing regime.

Boosting Liver Function

The liver is a clearing station for the body and filters out toxins. It also filters excess estrogen from the body, so it is an organ that needs to be kept in tip-top condition. Some useful liver herbs include:

- **DANDELION** has been used for many years as a general liver tonic, which makes it a useful menopause herb in an indirect way. The liver filters all that we eat and drink, as well as medications and hormones. When a women's hormone production level becomes unbalanced, the liver undergoes a great deal of stress.
- **MILK THISTLE** strengthens the liver.
- **YELLOW DOCK ROOT** helps metabolize estrogen out of the body, thus reducing fibroids.

Low Libido

Libido is affected by hormones, inclination, and how we feel about our partner. While herbs can't bring a sexual bloom to a boring or unhappy relationship, they can help to balance our hormones, which may lead to a satisfying sexual dalliance. Herbs that can improve the libido include:

- **DAMIANA** is a herb that is frequently used to stimulate the female libido.
- **SARSAPARILLA** is a herb that stimulates the production of testosterone and therefore improves a waning libido.

- **OAT STRAW** can be consumed in the form of oats for breakfast.
- **MACA ROOT** has been used for centuries in South America and is an adaptogen, meaning it helps to balance the body's hormonal system as needed.

> **WISE WOMAN WAYS**
>
> As part of the herbal tone to this chapter, I've includes some guidance on aromatherapy:
> - **Bloating:** grapefruit, lemon, and juniper
> - **Irritability:** geranium, bergamot, and clary sage
> - **Depression:** rose, clary sage, and bergamot
> - **Fatigue:** rosemary and basil
> - **Stress:** lavender and marjoram
> - **Headache:** peppermint, Roman chamomile, and lavender
> - **Cramps:** jasmine, Roman chamomile, cypress, and clary sage
> - **Heavy bleeding:** cypress, geranium, rose, yarrow, Roman chamomile, lavender, and lemon
>
> Use the oils on a warm compress or massage the abdomen or lower back with them. If you are using a hot water bottle to soothe the cramps, use warming oils such as sweet marjoram, or rosemary in a massage blend before using the hot water bottle. Or you might like to add a few drops to an already run bath. When I was in hospital having a mastectomy many moons ago, I had an electric burner by my bedside, where I constantly had geranium on the go to balance my hormones. It was very soothing, I can tell you—both for me and the nurses!

Heavy Bleeding

Heavy bleeding can be due to a number of factors, including menopause, endometriosis, polyps, fibroids, or pelvic inflammatory disease. A period is heavy if you have flooding; you bleed for more than eight days (month after month); you bleed so much that it is difficult for you to get on with your life; the bleeding is so heavy that you become anemic; and/or you have large clots for more than one or two days. You may find these herbs helpful for heavy bleeds:

- **WILD YAM** (progestogenic properties)
- **AGRIMONY**
- **CRAMP BARK** and **VALERIAN** (and for cramps)
- **LADY'S MANTLE** (and for cramps).
- **BIOFLAVONOIDS** strengthen capillaries and provide estrogenic factors that help decrease flooding. Plants containing bioflavonoids include dong quai, black cohosh, blue cohosh, unicorn root, false unicorn root, fennel, anise, sarsaparilla, and wild yam root. Generally, yellow, orange, and red vegetables and fruits are good sources of bioflavonoids.
- **RASPBERRY LEAF** is a nutritive estrogenic herb and astringent that works directly on the uterus, toning weakened muscles and relaxing uterine spasms.
- **SAGE** (blood clots in heavy bleed)
- **SHEPHERD'S PURSE** (often taken with yarrow) functions as a pituitary regulator with androgenic properties to normalize progesterone levels.
- **STINGING NETTLE**
- **VITEX AGNUS CASTUS** helps the body produce progesterone, which balances estrogen. It takes a couple of cycles to kick in and needs to be taken daily.
- **CINNAMON BARK** relieves uterine cramping and checks flooding.

- **WITCH HAZEL** fosters normal menstruation and has a tonic effect on the uterus.
- **MISTLETOE** and **BUTTERBUR** are good in combination for use in shrinking fibroids.
- Herbs that will increase your iron: Chickweed, kelp, burdock root, catnip, horsetail, Althea root, milk thistle seed, uva ursi, dong quai, black cohosh, echinacea, licorice, valerian, and sarsaparilla roots; and nettles, plantain leaf, fenugreek seed, and peppermint. Dandelion leaves and yellow dock root are excellent for flooding as they contain a bioavailable form of iron, which is lost in excessive flooding.

Heavy bleeding has always been an issue for me, especially in the first couple of days of my period, necessitating hourly visits to the loo and, if I'm away from home, regular pit stops between train, bus, car, or building. Now that I'm in the menopausal arena, I have what I call my Jerry Lewis run. On the morning of the second day of my period I can be prone to a flood first thing, leading to a sideways shuffle out of bed followed by a knock-kneed run to the loo.

> **WISE WOMAN WAYS**
> A herbal tea, or tisane, is a (hot or cold) herbal infusion made from the combination of boiling water and fresh or dried flowers, leaves, seeds, or roots. The tisane is then strained before drinking. The longer the infusion steeps, the stronger the qualities of the herb you drink. I'm having some flooding at the moment. In speaking to my homeopath, we discussed the differences between making herbal tea or taking a herbal tincture. The outcome of the conversation was that there's not much difference between the two.

However, making fresh herbal tea with dried herbs is much better than herbal tea bags.

I've chosen to drink a tea made up of a combination of ladies mantle and raspberry leaf (2 heaped teaspoons into a teapot and infused for 10 minutes). I drink this once a day, normally—three times a day when I'm bleeding, to lessen the flow (it works wonders). The tea tastes good, and I like the ritual of making this tea and sitting quietly to drink it.

Water Retention

Premenstrual time can make us look like barrage balloons, full of liquid, wind, and pee. The following herbs can lessen the water we hold in our bodies:

- **DANDELION** strengthens the liver and helps it process excess hormones.
- **CLEAVERS HERB** tincture tells the lymphatic tissues to get moving and is especially helpful for swollen, sore breasts.
- **EVENING PRIMROSE OIL** is an adaptogen and useful for fluid retention.

Headaches

For some women, periods bring on headaches. Chinese herbalists say headaches are caused by liver stress. Liver-strengthening herbs are dandelion, yellow dock, milk thistle seed, and burdock. The following herbs may also be helpful:

- **SAGE** offers relief from headaches.
- **SOY** is a phytoestrogen and can help with migraine headaches.
- **SKULLCAP** can ease pain and relieve muscle spasms.

- **EVENING PRIMROSE OIL** is an adaptogen and is useful for treating headaches.

Mood Swings

Tears on the pillow. Ax almost sunk into partner's head. The calamity of the vegetables boiling over. The panic attack in the grocery store. These are familiar to almost all menstruating women, I'm sure. The following herbs may help to soothe the furrowed brow:

- **EVENING PRIMROSE OIL** is an adaptogen and useful for mood swings, anxiety, and irritability.
- **SOY** is a phytoestrogen and can help with mood swings.
- **LICORICE ROOT** is a phytoestrogen and can help with mood swings and menopausal depression due to its activity on specific neurotransmitters.
- **OAT STRAW** strengthens the nerves and helps reduce emotional distress.
- **DAMIANA** can act as a mild antidepressant.
- **NETTLE** will strengthen the adrenals and ease anxiety.
- **TRUE UNICORN ROOT** is an estrogenic herb and provides a mild sedative action.
- **ASHWAGANDHA** is an adaptogen and is used as a herb for gentle relaxation and emotional balance.
- **RED CLOVER** grows naturally in Europe and Asia and is one of the premium sources of phytoestrogens, the weak plant estrogens that help balance estrogen levels in the body, thereby reducing menopausal symptoms. Studies on red clover show that it does seem to reduce symptoms of mood swings in menopause.
- **VITEX AGNUS CASTUS** is useful as a menopause herb as it alleviates the symptoms of depression.

- **MOTHERWORT** has a calming effect but does not make you drowsy.
- **BLACK COHOSH** is touted as a great reliever of anxiety and depression. Black cohosh may be taken up to twice a day for six months, but should not be taken for a longer period of time.
- **DONG QUAI** is nicknamed the "female ginseng" and contains phytoestrogens. Dong quai is a mild sedative that will help reduce mood swings and stress related to menopause. Dong quai is especially effective when used in combination with black cohosh.

WISE WOMAN WAYS

My garden is large and rural, although I live on the outskirts of a large city. I leave the beds to do their own thing (with a little pruning), and there are loads of plants in pots everywhere. I would love to grow herbs but don't, for two reasons. One is the number of slugs and snails, which insist on taking their package holidays throughout the year with us. Secondly, I get through the herbs too fast. So I have to confess to doing the modern Wise Woman thing and getting my fresh culinary herbs from our local organic greengrocer up the road, my medicinal tinctures from an organic herbalist, and my fresh dried herbs for tea from Neal's Yard in Covent Garden, London.

Insomnia

A few days before your monthly bleed, you may experience sleeplessness due to fluctuating hormones. They can also cause an increase in body temperature, causing insomnia.

- **OAT STRAW** in the form of a tincture or porridge promotes sound sleep. Try it an hour before you go to bed.
- **PASSIFLORA, HOPS, KAVA KAVA, WILD LETTUCE, LAVENDER, CHAMOMILE, VALERIAN ROOT,** and **PASSIONFLOWER** are traditional herbs for insomnia. They are best taken in tincture, capsule, or tea form. Put 1 cup of boiling water into a teapot and add 1 tsp. chamomile flowers, 1 tsp. hops, and 1 tsp. valerian root. Steep for 45 minutes and strain. Drink an hour before retiring.

Fatigue

I experience a drop in energy a couple of days before a period and during the first couple of days. You may find the following helps to boost your energy:

- **OAT STRAW** infusion builds energy and eases anxiety.
- **NETTLE** infusion increases energy without wiring your nerves. Nettle strengthens the adrenals, allowing you to tolerate more stress with less harm. The plants with the deepest green give you the most energy. Drink a daily cup of nettle infusion for fatigue.
- **GINSENG** strengthens the adrenal glands, increases immunity, boosts energy, and normalizes blood pressure. It can be used for treating mental and physical fatigue. Siberian ginseng has been shown to be somewhat more effective than the American variety. Asian ginseng is an adaptogen and helps the body resist stress and adapt to change.
- **SARSAPARILLA** can increase energy and overall feelings of vitality.
- **LICORICE** acts as a powerful adrenal stimulant and estrogenic herb. The effect on the adrenal gland is enhanced by adding Asian ginseng. It also blocks the activity of a specific

enzyme that subsequently increases the activity of cortisol (helpful for adrenal fatigue). NOTE: If you have high blood pressure, you need to be careful about the stimulating effect of licorice; however, if you have low blood pressure, licorice may be quite beneficial.

Constipation

It is important to prevent constipation as it can make hemorrhoids (piles) worse. Here are some herbs to try:

- **DANDELION** or **MALLOW** tea, made from the leaves of the plants, steeped in boiling water, and drunk daily can help treat constipation.
- **FENUGREEK, PSYLLIUM HUSKS,** and **LINSEEDS** (FLAXSEEDS) provide fiber, which bulks up the waste matter in the colon, helping the stools pass more easily.
- **SLIPPERY ELM** is an emollient herb, which means it lubricates the intestinal tract and soothes the mucous membranes of an irritated stomach, making it an ideal herb to use for constipation.
- **CASCARA SAGRADA, BARBERRY, CAYENNE, TURKEY RHUBARB**, and a number of other herbs are great for long-term constipation.
- **CAPE ALOE** is extracted from the outer skin of the aloe vera plant and is a strong laxative—only to be used very occasionally.

Add 3-4 drops of essential oils such as sweet orange, lemon, lime, grapefruit, or bergamot to your bath and relax in the warm water for a while; you could also use plenty of soap lather to massage your tummy gently in a clockwise direction.

Herbal Sources of Vitamins

- **VITAMIN B COMPLEX:** For healthy digestion, good liver function, emotional flexibility, less anxiety, and sound sleep. *Herbal sources:* Red clover blossoms, parsley leaf, and oatstraw.
- **VITAMIN B1** (thiamine): For emotional ease, strong nerves. *Herbal sources:* Peppermint, burdock, sage, yellow dock, alfalfa, red clover, fenugreek seeds, raspberry leaf, nettle, catnip, watercress, yarrow leaf/flower, and rose buds and hips.
- **VITAMIN B2** (riboflavin): For more energy, healthy skin. *Herbal sources:* Peppermint, alfalfa greens, parsley, echinacea, yellow dock, hops, dandelion root, ginseng, dulse, kelp, fenugreek seed, rose hips, and nettles.
- **VITAMIN B9** (folic acid): For calm nerves. *Herbal sources:* Leafy greens of nettles, alfalfa, parsley, sage, catnip, peppermint, plantain, comfrey, and chickweed.
- **VITAMIN B3** (niacin): For relief of anxiety and depression, decrease in headaches, and reduction of serum cholesterol levels. *Herbal sources:* Hops, raspberry leaf, red clover, slippery elm, echinacea, licorice, rose hips, nettle, alfalfa, and parsley.
- **BIOFLAVONOIDS:** For a healthy heart and to reduce menstrual bleeding, breast lumps, water retention, and anxiety. *Herbal sources:* Buckwheat greens, elderberries,

hawthorn fruits, rose hips, horsetail, shepherd's purse, and chervil.

- **CAROTENES:** For a well-lubricated vagina, protection against cancer, and healthy lungs and skin. *Herbal sources:* Peppermint, yellow dock, uva ursi, parsley, alfalfa, raspberry, nettles, dandelion greens, kelp, green onions, violet leaves, cayenne, paprika, lamb's quarters leaves, sage, chickweed, horsetail, black cohosh roots, and rose hips.
- **VITAMIN C COMPLEX:** For insomnia and fewer headaches, better resistance to infection, and easier emotions. Depleted by stress and aging. *Herbal sources:* Rose hips, yellow dock root, raspberry leaf, red clover, hops, pine needles, dandelion greens, alfalfa greens, echinacea, skullcap, plantain, parsley, cayenne, and paprika.
- **VITAMIN E:** For protection from cancer, fewer signs of aging, fewer wrinkles, moist vagina, strong heart, and freedom from arthritis. *Herbal sources:* Alfalfa, rosehips, nettles, dong quai, watercress, dandelion, seaweeds, and wild seeds of lamb's quarters and plantain.
- **ESSENTIAL FATTY ACIDS** (EFAS), including GLA, omega 6, and omega 3: For a healthy heart, strong nerves, well-functioning endocrine glands, and fewer wrinkles. All wild plants, but very few cultivated plants, contain EFAs; fresh purslane is notably high.
- **VITAMIN K:** For less menstrual flooding. *Herbal sources:* Nettle, alfalfa, kelp, and green tea.

WISE WOMAN WAYS

Herbal honeys are made by pouring honey over fresh herbs and allowing them to infuse over a period of several days to several months. As the herbs are infused with honey, the water-loving honey absorbs all the water-soluble oils of the herb. Here's how to create your herbal honey:

- Coarsely chop the dried herb of your choice (ginger and garlic should be used fresh). You could use sage, rose, mint, oregano, lemon verbena, lavender, fennel seeds, thyme, rosemary, marjoram, or lemon balm.
- Put chopped herb into a wide-mouthed jar, filling almost to the top. Pour pasteurized honey into the jar, working it into the herb with a wooden spoon. Fill the jar to the very top and cover tightly and label.

Your herbal honey is ready to use in as little as a day or two, but it will be more medicinal if allowed to sit for six weeks. Ways to use your herbal honey include spreading it on home-made bread or placing a tablespoonful (include herb as well as honey) into a mug of boiling water.

Herbal Sources of Minerals

- **CALCIUM:** For sound sleep, freedom from depression and headaches, less bloating, and fewer mood fluctuations. *Herbal sources:* Valerian, kelp, nettle, horsetail, peppermint, sage, uva ursi, yellow dock, chickweed, red clover, oat straw, parsley, black currant leaf, raspberry leaf, plantain leaf/seed, dandelion leaf, amaranth leaf/seed, and lamb's quarter leaf/seed.
- **CHROMIUM:** For less fatigue, fewer mood swings, stable blood sugar levels, and increased high-density lipoprotein (HDL), known as the "good" cholesterol.

Herbal sources: Oat straw, nettle, red clover tops, catnip, dulse, wild yam, yarrow, horsetail; roots of black cohosh, licorice, echinacea, valerian, and sarsaparilla.

- **COPPER:** For supple skin, healthy hair, calm nerves, less water retention, less menstrual flooding, and lower serum cholesterol. *Herbal sources:* Skullcap, sage, horsetail, and chickweed.

- **IODINE:** For fewer breast lumps, less fatigue, and stronger liver. *Herbal sources:* Kelp, parsley, celery, and sarsaparilla root.

- **IRON:** For fewer headaches, less menstrual flooding, better sleep, calmer nerves, more energy, and less dizziness. *Herbal sources:* Chickweed, kelp, burdock root, catnip, horsetail, Althea root, milk thistle seed, uva ursi, dandelion leaf/root; yellow dock, dong quai, black cohosh, echinacea, licorice, valerian, and sarsaparilla roots; and nettles, plantain leaf, fenugreek seed, and peppermint.

- **MAGNESIUM:** For deeper sleep, less anxiety, easier nerves, lower low-density lipoprotein (LDL), or "bad," cholesterol, more energy, and fewer headaches/migraines. *Herbal sources:* Oat straw, licorice, kelp, nettle, dulse, burdock root, chickweed, Althea root, horsetail, sage, raspberry leaf, red clover, valerian, yellow dock, dandelion greens, carrot tops, parsley leaf, evening primrose.

- **MOLYBDENUM:** For prevention of anemia. *Herbal sources:* Nettles, dandelion greens, sage, oat straw, fenugreek seeds, raspberry leaves, red clover blossoms, horsetail, chickweed, and kelp.

- **NICKEL:** For calmer nerves. *Herbal sources:* Alfalfa, red clover, oat straw, and fenugreek.

- **PHOSPHORUS:** For more energy. *Herbal sources:* Peppermint, yellow dock, milk thistle, fennel, hops, chickweed, nettle, dandelion, parsley, dulse, and red clover.
- **POTASSIUM:** For more energy, less water retention, easy weight loss, steady heart beat, and better digestion. *Herbal sources:* Sage, catnip, peppermint, skullcap, hops, dulse, kelp, red clover, horsetail, nettles, and plantain leaf.
- **SELENIUM:** For slower aging, strong immunity, less irritability, more energy, healthy hair/nails/teeth, and less cardiovascular disease. *Herbal sources:* Catnip, milk thistle seed, valerian root, dulse, black cohosh and ginseng roots; uva ursi leaf, hops flowers, kelp, raspberry leaf, rose buds and hips, hawthorn berries, fenugreek seed, roots of echinacea, sarsaparilla, and yellow dock.
- **SILICON:** For less irritable nerves. *Herbal sources:* Horsetail, dulse, echinacea, cornsilk, burdock, oat straw, licorice, chickweed, uva ursi, and sarsaparilla.
- **SULFUR:** For soft skin and glossy hair, healthy nerves, and strong liver. *Herbal sources:* Sage, nettles, plantain, and horsetail.
- **ZINC:** For slower aging, better digestion, stronger bones, healthy skin, cancer prevention, and increased sex drive. *Herbal sources:* Skullcap, sage, wild yam, chickweed, echinacea, nettles, dulse, milk thistle, and sarsaparilla.

WISE WOMAN WAYS

If you are on ANY medication, please consult a qualified medical herbalist[13] before taking herbs, as there can be distressing interactions between some pharmaceutical medications and herbal compounds.

MENSTRUFACT

The family of words that are related to the English word "menstruation" include mental, memory, meditation, mensurate, commensurate, meter, mother, mana, magnetic, mead, mania, man, and moon.

What Happens Next?

The use of herbs in Wise Woman healing, both internally and externally, is part of our sacred heritage. While flower essences aren't to be confused with herbs or essential oils, they too have their precious place in our life during the menstruation years. Read on to discover how you might use these gifts from nature.

CHAPTER 6

Using Flower Essences for Menstruation

From the beginning of time, nature has provided the means to heal on all levels. Flower essences have been used for centuries in Australia, South America, Asia, Egypt, South America, and India. They were also very popular in Europe in the Middle Ages. Hildegard von Bingen, a 12th-century visionary who wrote medicinal texts, and Paracelsus, a 15th-century physician and astrologer, both wrote how they used dew collected from flowering plants to treat health imbalances.

How Flower Essences Work

Flower essences are a form of vibrational medicine and act in a similar way to homeopathic remedies by working with subtle energy in the body. All living things, including our body and mind, are matter that is permeated by, and surrounded by, subtle energy. We could define subtle energy as the underpinning source feeding the well-being of our mind and body.

According to the concept of energy medicine, disease manifests in the physical body only after energy flow in the subtle body has been disturbed. Energy medicine has been long been practiced by civilizations such as India and China, and is gradually being integrated into Western healthcare. The energy field model used by these civilizations as part of their eclectic healthcare system, which includes acupuncture, moves away from the main idea that life evolves from a scientific blueprint, towards the concept that life circulates via electrical charges of energy known as *prana* or *chi*. In addition to this circulation of energy, there is a force field of energy permeating the human body called the aura, which can influence our well-being.

In order to rebalance the subtle body, we must administer energy that vibrates at frequencies beyond the physical plane. Just as we might heal the physical body through medical interventions, we need to heal the subtle body through vibrational interventions such as homeopathy, crystals, or flower essences.

Flower essences work by utilizing the essence's positive energy to transmute a negative state in living things, whether they are human, animal, or plant. Each flower used in a flower essence conveys a subtle energy pattern that is transferred to water during essence preparation. This preparation is then either used internally or externally for healing purposes.

From a spiritual perspective, flower essences address mental and emotional imbalances that, if left unresolved, could influence the wellness of the physical body. In effect, we "co-create" with the flower essences to alter our subtle energies when we use them for healing purposes. This change permeates our emotional and mental states and can also influence our physical well-being. The belief that we can heal ourselves is the basis of flower essence philosophy. Essences do not affect us biochemically, as does traditional allopathic medicine. They are water-based products that have no chemical or biological materials present other than water and alcohol preservatives.

Bach Flower Remedies

Dr. Edward Bach[14] studied medicine at University College Hospital in London, qualified in 1912, and became casualty medical officer at the hospital in 1913. He worked in general practice in London's famed medical sector Harley Street and as a bacteriologist and pathologist working on vaccines. In the course of his work, he came to question some of the tenets of early 20th-century medical practice. Bach believed that the illness-personality link was a product of unbalanced energetic patterns within the subtle body, and that illness was a reflection of disharmony between the physical personality and the Higher Self.

Bach took a post at the Royal London Homeopathic Hospital in 1919, during which time he noticed the parallels between his work on vaccines and the principles of homeopathy. Although his work up to this point had been with bacteria, he wanted to find healing modalities that would be less toxic and more in tune with the mind-body link. To this end, he began collecting plants in the hope of replacing the nosodes (homeopathic remedies prepared from infected tissues) with a series of gentler remedies.

In 1928, Bach acquired two wildflowers, impatiens and mimulus, which he homeopathically prepared and clinically used with excellent results. He soon understood that there was great healing power in flowers, and he gradually developed his own methods of preparing flower essences. In the early 1930s, Bach left his successful practice and began gathering wildflowers, which he developed into 38 flower remedies.

Instead of scientific methodology, he chose to rely on his intuitive gifts as a healer. He found that he could place the flowers of a particular species on the surface of a bowl of spring water for several hours in sunlight and obtain powerful vibrational tinctures. The subtle effects of sunlight charged the water with an energetic imprint of the flower's unique signature.

In 1934, Dr. Bach moved to Mount Vernon in Oxfordshire, England, and it was here, in the surrounding countryside, that he found the remaining flower remedies he sought, each aimed at a particular mental state or emotion. Bach's work was in tune with nature's own annual cycle. In spring and summer, he found the flowers he needed in the countryside and prepared individual flower remedies, then in winter, he helped and advised patients. He found that when he treated the feelings of his patients, their distress and physical discomfort would be alleviated to allow their natural healing to come through.

The 38 Bach Flower Remedies include:

agrimony	aspen
beech	centaury
cerato	cherry plum
chestnut bud	chicory
clematis	crab apple
elm	gentian
gorse	heather
holly	honeysuckle
hornbeam	impatiens
larch	mimulus
mustard	oak
olive	pine
red chestnut	rock rose
rock water	schleranthus
star of Bethlehem	sweet chestnut
vervain	vine
walnut	water violet
white chestnut	wild oat
wild rose	willow

Menstruation Issue	**Recommended Bach Flower Remedy**
Mood changes	scleranthus
Fear of pain	mimulus, rock rose
Impatience	impatiens
Feeling overwhelmed	elm
Worry, apprehension	white chestnut, red chestnut, aspen, larch
Feeling like an elephant!	crab apple
Depression	cherry plum, gentian, gorse, mustard, white chestnut, and wild rose

Fretful	agrimony
Fuzzy thinking, lack of concentration	crab apple, clematis
Indecisive, self-doubting	cerato, scleranthus, wild oat
Insomnia	holly, hornbeam, mustard, olive, white chestnut
Intolerant, critical, irritable	beech, holly, impatiens, rock water, vervain, vine, crab apple
Irrational without knowing why	cherry plum
Lack of confidence	centaury, larch, and mimulus
Panic	cherry plum, rock rose
Tired, drained	olive
Headache	aspen, vervain, white chestnut

I came to the Bach Flower Remedies about 25 years ago. A friend had a computer and photocopy shop, and I would sometimes help out. One day a nutritionist came in with a mound of copying to do, much of it related to flower essences. Being full of curiosity, I was reading as I was copying. It was like coming home. I learnt the remedies by using them on myself, and since those days all the remedies have been in my home ready to use with family, friends, animals, plants, clients, students, and myself.

Animals and young children respond particularly well to Bach Flower Remedies. I remember going to an animal sanctuary on the request of a student of mine who worked there. In a glass terrarium was a mother snake and several babies. Mum snake, bless her, had a cold and was coiled in a corner. I made up a remedy for the student to give to the mother snake, and within minutes she picked up and got right into a bit of family entwining! I've given remedies to cats following operations and dogs in crisis over fireworks night. I've also had lots of success giving remedies to babies and young children with sleep and behavioural issues at the parent's request.

I've found that it's important to use the remedy or remedies that resonate as the right ones at the gut level—however off the wall they might seem at the time. It's a good idea to carry Bach Flower Rescue Remedy as an emergency stress-buster. It's a mixture of rock rose, impatiens, clematis, star of Bethlehem, and cherry plum and works rapidly to calm the body.

Australian Bush Flower Essences

Since Dr. Bach created his flower essences in the 1930s, the issues we face in our lives have changed. As we came to the end of the 20th century and slipped into the 21st century, there was a growing need for flower essences that help people deal with the issues of today.

While many new flower essences have found their way to the commercial market, some of the most effective new flower essences come from Australian plants[15] as a result of the work of Ian White, a naturopath and fifth-generation Australian herbalist. Ian grew up in the Australian bush. His grandmother, like her mother before her, specialized in using Australian plants and, when he was a young boy, would often take him bush walking to learn the healing qualities of plants and flowers. He learned a profound respect for nature through her and went on to become a practitioner and a pioneer working with and researching the rare remedial qualities of Australian native plants. Australia is relatively unpolluted, has some of the world's oldest plants, and metaphysically has a wise, old energy.

The 65 Australian Bush Essences include:

alpine mint bush	angelsword
banksia robur	bauhinia
billy goat plum	black-eyed Susan

bluebell

boab

boronia

bottlebrush

bush fuchsia

bush gardenia

bush iris

crowea

dagger hakea

dog rose

dog rose of wild forces

five corners

flannel flower

freshwater mangrove

fringed violet

green spider orchid

grey spider flower

gymea lily

hibbertia

illawarra flame tree

isopogon

jacaranda

kangaroo paw

kapok bush

little flannel flower

macrocarpa

mint bush

mountain devil

mulla mulla

old man banksia

paw paw

peach-flowered tea tree

philotheca

pink mulla mulla

red grevillea

red helmet orchid

red lily

red suva frangipani

rough bluebell

she oak

silver princess

slender rice flower

Southern Cross

spinifex

sturt desert pea

sturt desert rose

sundew

sunshine wattle

tall mulla mulla

tall yellow top

turkey bush

waratah

wedding bush

wild potato bush

wisteria

yellow cowslip orchid

Menstruation Issue	Recommended Australian Bush Essence
Apprehensive, anxious	Tall mulla mulla, dog rose, and illawarra flame tree
Constipation	Bauhinia, bottlebrush, flannel flower, and bluebell
Depression	Waratah and tall yellow top
Self-doubting	Five corners, kapok bush, red grevillea, and bush fuchsia
Insomnia	Boronia, grey spider flower, black-eyed Susan, and crowea
Intolerant, critical, irritable	Yellow cowslip orchid, mountain devil, and black-eyed Susan
Lack of confidence	Five corners and kapok bush
Lack of sexual interest	Billy goat plum
Mental and emotional exhaustion	Alpine mint bush, banksia robur, macrocarpa
Panic	Grey spider flower, dog rose of the wild forces
Resentful	Dagger hakea
Tired, drained	Old man banksia
Worry	Crowea
Physical exhaustion	Marcrocarpa
Headache	Black-eyed Susan

The Australian Bush Flower Essences found me through a book—or rather that's how I remembered them again. While I have never been to Australia, there is some link to this wild country in my soul. I've used them increasingly over the years. I have the full range of bush essences, which I often blend with the Bach Flower

Remedies. I find the Australian Bush Flower Essences very profound in their action.

> **WISE WOMAN WAYS**
>
> When using flower essences, it's important to use them in an integrated way. Don't just take them mindlessly. When I take a remedy, I consider why I'm taking it and what I can do to support myself in other ways. For example, if I'm taking a mixture for anger, I ask myself what or who is my anger directed at. What can I do to help externalize this feeling? What is it about? I might choose to journal my thoughts and feelings or talk them through with someone, taking the remedies as I consciously work through my issue.

How to Mix and Use Remedies

Here are a variety of ways you can use the remedies:

Combination mixtures

Using a blend of Bach and Australian Bush Flower Essences, you can make up these remedies. Take them either directly from the bottle or moisten your lips. NOTE: BF = Bach Flowers and ABFE = Australian Bush Flower Essences

Menstruation State	Recommended Remedy
Fear of pain	Mimulus (BF), rock rose (ABFE)
Impatience	Impatiens (BF)
Feeling overwhelmed	Elm (BF)
Worry	White chestnut (BF), red chestnut (BF), aspen (BF), larch (BF), tall mulla mulla (ABFE), dog rose (ABFE), illawarra

	flame tree (ABFE), crowea (ABFE), and agrimony (BF)
Lack of confidence	Centaury (BF), larch (BF), mimulus (BF), five corners (ABFE), and kapok bush (ABFE)
Panic	Cherry plum (BF), rock rose (BF), grey spider flower (ABFE), and dog rose of the wild forces (ABFE)
Tired, drained	Olive (BF), old man banksia (ABFE), and marcrocarpa (ABFE)
Self-doubting	Five corners (ABFE), kapok bush (ABFE), red grevillea (ABFE), cerato (BF), and wild oat (BF)
Mental and emotional exhaustion	Alpine mint bush (ABFE), banksia robur (ABFE), and macrocarpa (ABFE)
Anxiety	Aspen (BF), mimulus (BF), larch (BF), rock rose (BF), crowea (ABFE), and illawarra flame tree (ABFE)
Irritability	Beech (BF), vervain (BF), black-eyed Susan (ABFE), and yellow cowslip orchid (ABFE)

Internal

Flower essences can be taken orally for acute cases by putting 2–3 drops of the stock bottle essence under the tongue. They can be taken longer term by taking 6 drops from a dropper bottle that contains stock essence plus water. To make up a remedy:

1. Fill a 20ml glass dropper bottle with tap or filtered water to a finger width beneath the neck of the bottle.

2. Choose your remedy (you can use a mixture of Australian Bush Flower Essences and Bach Flower Remedies for up to six remedies). Put 2 drops from the stock bottle into the dropper bottle.

3. If you are a Reiki practitioner, you might like to perform Reiki on the bottle.

4. Take 4 drops under the tongue, 4 times daily. Alternatively you can put the remedies in tea, coffee, fizzy drinks, and so on. If you are taking a made-up remedy, you might have 4 drops, 4 times daily for a period of one month or lunar cycle. Note: Putting the drops into a hot drink has the advantage of evaporating the alcohol. This is sometimes recommended to people who dislike the alcohol content or who are too sensitive to alcohol to take remedies containing it, such as those with adrenal issues.

Because of the dynamic nature of awakening and going to sleep at night, the most important times to take the remedy is immediately upon waking and before going to sleep. The other two times may be before lunch and around 6pm.

- INHALING: Put two drops of your chosen essence in the palm of your hands, rub them together, and inhale from them.
- MEDITATION: One of the most powerful ways to use the essences is to take a few drops just before meditating.
- IN FOOD: When you make nourishing food for yourself, add your remedy to the food, either straight from the stock bottle or from your dropper bottle mixture.

WISE WOMAN WAYS

I find that taking the remedies is a multilayered opportunity for personal growth. When I feel distressed, I want the feelings to go away. I don't like feeling uncomfortable. I want to feel good. However, it isn't helpful to use the remedies as a "band-aid." Yes, the feelings may ease, but they may return again. Let's use anxiety as an example. Very often anxiety is the "acceptable face" we show the world. Anxiety, however, often covers up a range of other emotions that maybe aren't quite as "acceptable." Only the other day, I experienced feelings of being overwhelmed and anxious due to external pressures. I took myself off, did some relaxation exercises, a few stretches, and screamed into a cushion for good measure. There was the anger my anxiety had been holding down. So I took a remedy for the anger and helped myself through the blip.

WISE WOMAN WAYS

If your boobs feel tender, sprinkle several drops of she oak on a damp, cool flannel and place on the sensitive area.

External

- COMPRESS: This can be especially useful for sore places, such as the breasts or lower back. To prepare a flower essence compress, fill a bowl with warm or cold water. Add 4 drops of each chosen flower essence (and 1–2 drops of appropriate essential oil if you like) to the water. Soak the flannel or cotton wool in the water, wring out, and lay it on the affected area. Repeat until relief is felt.

- BATHING: Run a bath. The water needs to be at body temperature or a little warmer. Add 1–2 drops of your chosen essence. Essential oils can also be added after the water is run. Get into the bath and relax for 20 minutes. Rest afterwards. If you don't want to have a bath, bathing the feet and/or hands is also an effective way to take essences in through the skin.

- BODY SPRAY: Adding essential oils to a body spray brings not only added healing benefits but also a wonderful uplifting smell. Lighter oils, such as lavender or lemongrass, work best. To prepare a flower essence spray, fill a 50–125ml glass spray bottle with spring water. Add 3–4 drops of essential oil and 3 drops of each chosen flower essence. Shake the bottle to activate the essences. Spray twice daily, or as required.

- CHAKRA POINTS: With minimal knowledge of the chakra system, the seven wheel-shaped energy centers in the body, you can apply flower essences to a chakra area either directly from the stock bottle or take internally:

Chakra	Recommended Australian and Bach Flower Remedies
FIRST: Root (base) chakra	Waratah, red lily (disconnection), sundew (indecisive), grey spider (panic), macrocarpa (exhaustion), rock rose (panic), clematis (ungrounded), and hornbeam (mental exhaustion)
SECOND: Sacral (spleen) chakra	Turkey bush (creativity), billy goat plum (releases shame), spinifex

	(cleansing), and she oak (hormonal imbalance)
THIRD:	
Solar plexus	Old man banksia (counteracts weariness), macrocarpa (energy), crowea (releases worry), wild potato bush (releases feeling physically encumbered, weighted down), banksia robur (lethargy), cerato (strength to trust one's own judgment), and larch (lack of self-confidence)
FOURTH:	
Heart	Bush fuchsia (speaking your true essence), crowea (worry), flannel flower (intimacy), sturt desert pea (emotional pain), holly (blocked love), and gorse (despair)
FIFTH:	
Throat	Turkey bush (creative blocks)
SIXTH:	
Third-eye (brow)	Bush iris (clears blocks relating to grounding and trust), bush fuscia (intuition), and isopogon (memory)
SEVENTH:	
Crown	Red lily (disconnection), sundew (indecision), and wild oat (reconnecting)

- CREAM/LOTION: If what you need is just for now, put some cream in your hand, add the required stock essences drops, and mix before applying. To prepare a flower essence cream, fill a glass jar with 50g cream. You can use your favorite moisturizer as a base, but avoid any strongly scented creams. Add 4 drops of each chosen essence (up to four essences). Mix with a wooden stick or stiff drinking straw. You can add 1–2 drops of an essential oil to the cream to enhance its healing properties. Apply to the area twice daily, or as required.
- HEALING: Put the remedy on your hands before doing energy work such as Reiki, Wiccan, or shamanic practices on yourself.
- MASSAGE: Mixing essences in massage oil can greatly enhance your mood. Put 4 drops of essential oil, 1–2 drops of relevant flower essence, and 50ml of jojoba oil into a glass bottle. Mix and use immediately. Recommended oils: rose, ylang ylang, neroli, or lavender.
- TO ENHANCE BODYWORK: Flower essences are powerful tools when used in conjunction with acupuncture, energy work, massage, craniosacral therapy, or chiropractic treatments. Taking a few drops of flower essences before, during, and/or after a treatment helps the body "hold" positive adjustments by assisting the nervous system with repatterning as well as releasing the emotional/mental blocks.
- SUBTLE ENERGY MASSAGE: Place a few drops of your chosen flower essence on your hands and give yourself a subtle energy massage:

　　Keep your hands about 2 inches away from your body. Move your right hand from the heart area down the inside of your left arm and up the outside. Swap sides and do the same for the other arm.

Move your hands over the heart area, up over the head to the neck, and round to under the chin. Move down to under the breast area, round to the back (kidney area), and down over the buttocks and the back of the legs, imagining the movement going under the feet.

Return your hands to the heart area and move both hands down over the torso and down the front of both legs, imagining the movement going under the feet.

- ROOMS: You could put a flower essence mixture in a bowl of water on the mantelpiece or table, or add your chosen oils to your burner along with 4 drops of flower essence. Another idea is to make up a spray as in the instructions for creating a body spray above and use on bedding or in a room.

MENSTRUFACT

In 1946, Walt Disney made a movie about menstruation called "The Story of Menstruation." It is believed to be the first film to use the word "vagina."

What Happens Next?

While flower essences can contribute to improving our mindset, we can also develop the habit of relaxation and meditation as a useful mind-body skill. It can also enhance chakra healing, ritual, and quartz crystal healing. Curious? Turn to the page, gentle reader.

CHAPTER 7

Relaxation and Meditation

L earning to relax on a regular basis will not only calm your mind but will ease PMS and bleed discomfort. When we are in pain, we tend to tense our mind and body, which makes any discomfort worse. Learning to relax throughout your monthly cycle will make relaxation come easier during the bleeding time.

Learning to relax will help your body:

- increase the hormones serotonin and melatonin (which control relaxation and the sleep/wake cycle);
- produce endorphins (the hormone that reduces pain).

WISE WOMAN WAYS

How often is your period a nuisance? An inconvenience? To what extent do you shrug off your emotional sensitivity, intuition, or tiredness at this time? How much do you allow work, family, commitments—life—to get in the way of self-nourishment at any time during the month and at moontime? It took me many moons to learn to listen to myself as I approached my monthly bleed. In some ways it was my excuse to stop. I know now I don't need an excuse. I can stop when I'm not bleeding if I choose.

You could record any of the following relaxations or visualizations to reuse or ask someone to talk you through them.

Progressive Muscular Relaxation (PMR)

One of the most simple and easily learned techniques for relaxation is Progressive Muscle Relaxation (PMR), a widely used procedure today that was originally developed by American physician Edmund Jacobson in the 1920s.[16] The PMR procedure teaches you to relax your muscles through a two-step process coordinated with your inhale and exhale breaths. First, you breathe in and deliberately tighten up certain muscle groups to gain familiarity with how your muscles feel when tense. Then you exhale and let go of the tension in your muscles and focus your attention on noticing how the muscles feel now, in their relaxed state. By practicing daily throughout the month, you will be well versed in using the technique by the time you menstruate.

PMR Script

Find a comfortable place to sit, away from interruptions. Feel the chair support your body. Your feet are firmly on the floor, and your hands are resting lightly on your thighs. Take a deep breath and exhale completely.

- Bring your awareness down to your right foot. Breathe in and curl your toes under your right foot as tight as you can. Hold your breath, keeping the foot tight and feeling the tension. Now exhale, letting the toes go. Feel the relaxation in your feet and toes.
- Now, breathe in and curl your toes under on your left foot as tight as you can. Holding your breath, hold the toes tight and feel the tension. Exhale and let go of the muscles in your toes. Feel the relaxation in your feet and toes.
- Breathe in and tighten the muscles in your right foot by splaying your foot out. Hold your breath and hold your foot tight. Feel the tension. Now exhale and let go of the

muscles in the foot. Feel the relaxation in the muscles in your foot and toes.

- Now breathe in and tighten the muscles in your left foot by splaying your foot out. Hold your breath and hold the muscles tight. Feel the tension. Exhale and let the foot go. Feel the relaxation in the muscles in your foot and toes. Take a deep breath and exhale completely.

- Breathe in and tighten the front of the right leg by pointing your foot away from you, so that it is almost parallel with your leg. Hold your breath and hold the right leg tight. Now exhale and let the foot go. Feel the relaxation in the muscles in your leg, foot, and toes.

- Now breathe in and tighten the front of the left leg by pointing your foot away from you, so that it is almost parallel with your leg. Hold your breath, holding the left leg tight. Now exhale and let the foot go. Feel the relaxation in the muscles in your leg, foot, and toes.

- Breathe in and tighten the back of the right leg by flexing your foot upwards, stretching from your heel down. Hold your breath and hold the right leg tight. Now exhale and let the foot go. Feel the relaxation in the muscles in your leg, foot, and toes.

- Now breathe in and tighten the back of the left leg by flexing your foot upwards, stretching from your heel down. Hold your breath, holding the left leg tight. Now exhale and let the foot go. Feel the relaxation in the muscles in your leg, foot, and toes. Inhale deeply and exhale completely.

- Breathe in and tighten the muscles in your right thigh while pressing your knee down into the floor. Hold the breath and keep the muscles tight. Now exhale and let the muscles go. Relax the muscles in your right thigh. Relax the muscles in your calves, feet, and toes.

- Now breathe in and tighten all the muscles in your left thigh while pressing your knee down into the floor. Hold your breath and hold the muscles tight. Now exhale, letting the muscles go. Feel the relaxation in the muscles in your left thigh. Feel the relaxation in the muscles in your calves, feet, and toes. Keep breathing. We often hold our breath when we have tension in the body. Inhale deeply and exhale completely.

- Breathe in and tighten the muscles in your bottom by clenching your buttocks together. Hold your breath and clench the buttocks. Now exhale and release the buttocks. Feel the relaxation in the muscles in your buttocks and thighs. Feel the relaxation in the muscles in your calves, feet, and toes.

- Breathe in and tighten the muscles in your stomach by drawing in your stomach. Hold your breath and hold the muscles tight. Now exhale and release the muscles. Feel the relaxation in the muscles in your stomach and your buttocks. Feel the relaxation in the muscles in your thighs. Feel the relaxation in the muscles in your calves, feet, and toes. You're breathing deeply and easily.

- Breathe in and tighten the muscles in your chest. Hold your breath, keeping your chest muscles tight. Now release the muscles as you exhale. Feel the relaxation in the muscles in your chest and stomach. Feel the relaxation in the muscles in your buttocks and thighs. Feel the relaxation in the muscles in your calves, feet, and toes. Take a deep breath and exhale completely, feeling even more relaxed.

- Breathe in and tighten the muscles in your shoulders by

pulling them up and forward. Hold your breath and hold the muscles tight. Now exhale and let the muscles go. Feel the relaxation in the muscles in your shoulders, chest, and stomach. Feel the relaxation in the muscles in your buttocks and thighs. Feel the relaxation in the muscles in your calves, feet and toes.

- Now breathe in and tighten the muscles in your shoulders by pulling them back. Hold your breath and tighten the muscles. Now exhale and let the muscles go. Feel the relaxation in the muscles in your shoulders, chest, and stomach. Feel the relaxation in the muscles in your buttocks and thighs. Feel the relaxation in the muscles in your calves, feet and toes. Breathe deeply and exhale completely.

- Breathe in and tighten the muscles in your right hand, making it into a fist. Hold your breath and hold the muscles tightly. Now exhale and let the hand go. Feel the relaxation in the muscles in your right hand and shoulders. Feel the relaxation in the muscles in your chest and stomach. Feel the relaxation in your buttocks and thighs. Feel the relaxation in your calves, feet and toes.

- Now breathe in and tighten the muscles in your left hand, making it into a fist. Hold your breath and hold the muscles tightly. Now exhale and let the hand go. Feel the relaxation in the muscles in your left hand and shoulders. Feel the relaxation in the muscles in your chest and stomach. Feel the relaxation in your buttocks and thighs. Feel the relaxation in your calves, feet and toes. Take in a breath and exhale completely.

- Breathe in and tighten the muscles in your right arm by tightening the biceps and lower arm together, but without the hand. Hold your breath and hold the muscles tight.

Now exhale and let them go. Feel the relaxation in your right arm, hand, and shoulders. Feel the relaxation in your chest and stomach. Feel the relaxation in your buttocks and thighs. Feel the relaxation in your calves, feet, and toes.

- Now breathe in and tighten the muscles in your left arm by tightening the biceps and lower arm together, but without the hand. Hold your breath and hold the muscles tight. Now exhale and let them go. Feel the relaxation in your left arm, hand, and shoulders. Feel the relaxation in your chest and stomach. Feel the relaxation in your buttocks and thighs. Feel the relaxation in your calves, feet, and toes. Feel yourself becoming more and more relaxed. Breathe deeply. Exhale completely.

- Now for a second time, breathe in and tighten the muscles in your shoulders. Hold your breath and hold the muscles tight. Now exhale and relax them. Feel the relaxation in the muscles in your shoulders, arms, and hands. Feel the relaxation in your chest and stomach. Feel the relaxation in your buttocks and thighs. Feel the relaxation in your calves, feet, and toes. Breathing deeply and easily.

- Now breathe in and tighten all the muscles in your neck. Stretch your head up, as if your chin could touch the ceiling. Then bend your head forward until your chin reaches your chest. Holding your breath, make the neck muscles very tight. Now exhale, letting go of all the muscles in your neck, shoulders, arms, and hands. Feel the relaxation in your chest and stomach. Feel the relaxation in your buttocks and thighs. Feel the relaxation in your calves, feet, and toes. You're breathing deeply and easily.

- Now, breathe in and tighten the muscles around your mouth and jaw by pressing your lips together and clenching your teeth. Holding your breath, hold the muscles tight. Now exhale and release the muscles. Feel the relaxation in the muscles in your mouth and jaw, your neck, shoulders, arms, and hands. Feel the relaxation in your chest and stomach. Feel the relaxation in your buttocks and thighs. Feel the relaxation in your calves, feet, and toes.

- Now breathe in and tighten the muscles in your forehead and scalp by raising your eyebrows as if they could disappear. Hold your breath and hold them tightly. Now exhale, letting them go. Feel the relaxation in the muscles around your mouth and jaw, your neck, shoulders, arms, and hands. Feel the relaxation in your chest and stomach. Feel the relaxation in your buttocks and thighs. Feel the relaxation in your calves, feet, and toes.

- Now breathe in and tighten the muscles in your face by screwing all the muscles up together. Hold your breath and hold the muscles tightly. Now exhale and let them go. Feel the relaxation in the muscles in your face, around your mouth and jaw. Feel the relaxation in the muscles in your neck, shoulders, arms, and hands. Feel the relaxation in your chest and your stomach. Feel the relaxation in your buttocks and thighs. Feel the relaxation in your calves, feet, and toes. Breathe in deeply and exhale completely.

- Now allow your mind to slowly scan your body from your head to toes, to be certain that there's no tension lingering in any muscles anywhere. And if you find any tension, focus your mind on letting go in that remaining part of you completely. You are now feeling completely relaxed from head to toe. You are more relaxed than you have been in a long while. Enjoy this time of deep relaxation. When you feel ready, open your eyes.

WISE WOMAN WAYS

Journaling your way through menstruation can be incredibly helpful. I've used journaling throughout my adult life—when I had breast cancer, through relationship difficulties, family issues, and work crisis. All you need is paper and pen. Your command of English doesn't matter—only your intent to externalize your thoughts and feelings. No one else need read your words or gaze on your doodling. Journaling has helped me work through problems and externalize difficult personal thoughts I wouldn't dream of telling anyone.

Create Your Special Place

The purpose of this visualization is to help you imagine in your mind's eye a special place where you feel safe, comfortable, and relaxed in order to let go and invite the wisdom from your inner wise woman during menstruation time. This place might be somewhere you know well or somewhere you create.

Close your eyes and take several slow, deep breaths. Now imagine a place where you feel completely safe, comfortable, and peaceful. It might be real or imaginary. Allow your special place to take shape visually through, colors, textures, and shapes. Listen to the sounds of your special place—water, music, animals, or the sounds of nature. You may feel a light wind touch your face or warm sun soothing your skin. You may feel grass between your toes, soft sand beneath your feet, or the support of a comfortable chair. Pick up a favorite object from your special place and use your fingertips to explore it. Take in a deep breath and notice all the rich fragrances around you—the scent of a flower, the tang of sea air, or the aroma of a special food you enjoy.

Relax into the serenity, comfort, and safety of your special place, breathing easily and deeply. As you inhale, visualize your breath going down to your belly. Visualize a light surrounding you that protects and nourishes you. Every part of your mind and body is filled with this powerful light. Feel it move deeper and deeper into every cell and organ, cleansing, opening, and balancing you. You are completely safe and loved. Your mind becomes calm and clear, and a feeling of renewed peace and strength fills you. Say to yourself: "I am safe. I am well. I am loved. As I move through my moon time, my power as a woman grows ever more profound." You feel peaceful and easy in your special place—a place that is always here. You know it's a place you can visit anytime, where you can experience this healing energy. When you are ready to return, take a deep breath and exhale fully. Open your eyes and spend a few moments enjoying this relaxed and comfortable feeling.

WISE WOMAN WAYS

Sit in a meditation position and practice the Yoni mudra (gesture) by bringing your fingers together into an almond shape, stretching the thumbs upwards and pointing the rest of the fingers downwards, keeping the center of your hands at the level of your spleen chakra. Do this for five minutes in the morning and evening, two days before your period, during your period, and two days after.

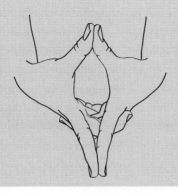

Relaxation Through
Better Breathing

There are two types of breathing: chest and abdominal (belly). Chest breathing is shallow, irregular, and fast, and the body does not receive the correct amount of oxygen. A tipoff to this is that a person will continually sigh, as a means of getting extra oxygen into the system, which provides short-term relief. This type of pattern often causes a person to hold their breath, hyperventilate, and experience shortness of breath. On top of this, the stress response will be activated hence more anxiety, and more shallow breathing. This type of breathing is also associated with mouth breathing, which the body immediately associates with stress. When you are stressed, your breathing becomes shallow. Breathing through the nose automatically soothes the system and leads to fuller belly breathing.

The other type of breathing is abdominal, or belly, breathing. Belly breathing is the way we are supposed to breathe, and it is a sign of health. Just watch a newborn baby breathing and you will see; it is adults who forget how to do this. As you inhale slowly and deeply through your nose, your lungs fill and expand with energizing oxygen (but the shoulders stay relaxed and the neck long), and as breath moves down into the body your diaphragm (solar plexus) simultaneously expands like a bell jar, pushing downwards into the abdominal cavity, giving the organs a nice massage and naturally causing the belly to push out. Then, as you exhale, the breath rises, as the belly button comes in toward the spine, the diaphragm relaxes, and the chest expands as the lungs deflate. Breathing in this way ensures that the lungs completely inflate then deflate, moving more oxygen into the body and, even more important, allowing carbon dioxide gas to completely be expelled from the lungs. Most people only use a fraction of their lung capacity, which leads to energy problems.

Abdominal breathing

Abdominal breathing can be very soothing because it slows you down. It is also efficient, as it ensures that a good supply of oxygen is reaching your brain. Check your breathing pattern by putting one hand on your chest and one hand on your stomach. If your lower hand moves and your top hand does not, you are doing abdominal breathing. But if your top hand moves and your bottom one does not, you are doing chest breathing.

You're going to inhale through your nose and exhale out of your mouth. Your exhalation needs to be longer than your inhalation. To slow your exhalation down, let your breath gently out, just enough to flicker a candle (purse your lips).

- Lay down flat and place your hands fingertip to fingertip, with your middle fingers meeting at your belly button.
- As you inhale through your nose, push your belly up and feel your fingertips expand. Rest a beat, before exhaling slowly through your mouth. Rest a beat before inhaling again and feel your belly rise. Repeat this cycle five times.
- Now place your hands under the breast area of each side of your body, which is the rib area.
- As you inhale through your nose, expand your ribs and feel your hands push out. Rest a beat, before exhaling slowly through your mouth. Rest a beat before inhaling again and feel your ribs expand. Repeat this cycle five times.
- Now you are going to do a complete breathing cycle, inhaling deeply from the belly and ribcage and exhaling completely.
- As you inhale through your nose for a count of five, push your belly up and expand your ribs. Rest a beat, before exhaling slowly through your mouth for a count of six. Rest a beat before inhaling again and feel your belly rise and your ribs expand. Repeat this cycle five times.

The more you practice abdominal breathing, the easier it will become. Eventually, you will be able to do it anywhere—sitting, standing, or lying down.

WISE WOMAN WAYS

Incredibly easy ways to chill:

- Go for a walk with no aim in mind, nothing to do, and no money on you to buy anything (apart from maybe a cup of tea or coffee!).
- Tuck yourself up in a quiet and comfortable place and go to sleep in the middle of the day.
- Indulge in a spell of comfort food, such as mashed potato, tomato soup, hot chocolate... well, you know the kind of thing.
- Buy something you have always wanted, can afford, and is a total waste of time and money—but it makes you incredibly happy.
- Lay in the grass watching the clouds through sleepy eyes.
- Lay on the beach with closed eyes, listening to the surf and the muted sounds of people around you.
- Lay under a tree.
- Paddle along the seashore's edge—as far as you can, as long as you like.
- Take a long walk by a long river.

Body Scan

Sit or lay down in a comfortable place where you won't be disturbed and close your eyes. Take in a slow, deep breath through your nose and exhale completely. And again. Allow your body to become comfortable as you breathe deeply and easily.

- Place your awareness in your forehead and scalp. Allow any tension in the forehead and scalp to drain over the back of the head and out of the base of your neck into infinity. You're breathing easily and deeply. Releasing and relaxing. Your eyes are gently closed. Ease away the frown. Wiggle your jaw from side to side to loosen the tension. Your tongue should be behind your lower teeth. You're breathing easily and deeply.
- Focus your awareness on your right shoulder and arm. Allow any tension in the right shoulder and arm to drain down the arm. Down, down, down the arm, out the fingers, and into infinity.
- Focus your awareness on your left shoulder and arm. Allow any tension in the left shoulder and arm to drain down the arm. Down, down, down the arm, out the fingers, and into infinity. You're breathing easily and deeply. Releasing and relaxing.
- Focus on the chest area. Feel the chest area opening and expanding. You're breathing easily and deeply.
- Focus on the stomach. Allow the stomach to relax. Releasing and relaxing.
- Focus your awareness on the back area. Upper back, middle back, and lower back. Allow any tension in the back area to slide down the spine. Down, down, down the spine, out the base of the spine, into infinity. You're breathing easily and deeply. Releasing and relaxing.
- Focus your attention on your right hip and leg. Allow any tension in the right hip and leg to drain down the leg. Down, down, down the leg, out the toes, into infinity.
- Focus your attention on your left hip and leg. Allow any tension in the left hip and leg to drain down the leg.

Down, down, down the leg, out the toes, into infinity. Releasing and relaxing.

- You feel completely relaxed from head to toe—more relaxed than you have been in a long while.

MENSTRUFACT

Orgasms, whether done through self-pleasure or intercourse, are a natural alternative to relieving menstrual cramps. Masters and Johnston reported that many women masturbate to relieve menstrual cramps, finding that orgasms increased the rate of blood flow and reduced cramping and backache. Orgasms cause the uterus to flex and contract, helping ease the pain and heaviness by facilitating blood flow, lessening the congested feeling within the pelvic area. Endorphins are also released after an orgasm and help the body to relax, temporarily relieving menstrual cramps.

What Happens Next?

Now that you feel more chilled, you have the ideal setting for healing on a subtle level. Let's find out how you can use chakra healing for a positive menstruation cycle.

CHAPTER 8

Chakra Healing

Think of yourself as an eclectic energy field of mind, body, and spirit—mind, with its intellect and emotions; the physical body; and the elusive spirit. Spiritual energy is less tangible, yet it permeates and underpins all the other energy fields. In addition to healing the mind and body during menstruation, we need to look at nourishing the energetic body that is part of our spiritual nature.

To grasp spiritual energy, we need to have some concept of the divine or the sacred. These two words could be defined as the infinite, the everlasting, God, Goddess, or universal energy. We may reflect that our human connection to the sacred is through our sense of spirituality, like an umbilical cord.

Our awareness of our spirituality, our connection to the divine, develops throughout our lifetime (or several). Metaphorically, you might consider your spirituality as a flame deep within you that burns brighter as you become more conscious.

> **WISE WOMAN WAYS**
> When I teach students about energetic anatomy, I explain it this way. Imagine you are a ball of light. This is your eternal flame, your link with the sacred, your spiritual self. In order for its brightness and connectedness to grow, you need to become increasingly aware of the defenses it has around it that dim its glow—defenses such as ego, anger, fear, and so on.

As you become more aware of yourself and work to let go of the mindsets that hold you back, more of these defenses will begin to fall away, allowing the ball of light to burn brighter still, increasing your connectedness to the sacred.

Imagine covering this ball of light in something like a loose-weave cloth. You can see the cloth, but because the weave is so loose, you can also see the glow of the ball through the cloth. This cloth represents your energetic anatomy, your auric field and chakra system. Energetic anatomy isn't a physical thing; it's a subtle energy manifestation and is as important as your physical anatomy. The energy field is like a multi-gateway system, through which you give and receive mental, emotional, physical, and spiritual energy. The more your ball glows and grows, the more the weave of your energy field expands. The development of your energetic anatomy and the development of your ball of light become increasingly one and the same.

The chakra system is part of your energy anatomy system and consists of several major chakras and many minor chakras. The word *chakra* is a Sanskrit word, meaning "vortex" or "wheel." These chakras aren't on the physical body but on the etheric body (part of your auric energy field). A major chakra resembles a spinning wheel. When balanced, it spins appropriately. If the chakra is blocked, the spin may be slower, counter-clockwise or static. When overstimulated, the chakra may be spinning too fast.

Each chakra has a relationship to our physical body, as well as to psychological mindsets. Our chakra system evolves as we grow older. This chapter will help you engage with chakra healing, as you travel through your monthly cycle.

The Chakra System

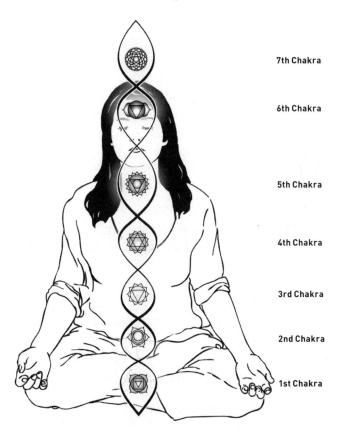

7th Chakra

6th Chakra

5th Chakra

4th Chakra

3rd Chakra

2nd Chakra

1st Chakra

Grounding Yourself

Before starting to perform any type of chakra healing, it is important to ground yourself. Grounding allows you to remain firmly connected to the earth by perceiving yourself anchored by roots that extend down to the core of the earth via your root chakra, for example. It prevents you from feeling "floaty" or "spaced out."

A grounding exercise

Sit or stand with eyes closed and observe your breathing for a few minutes. Visualize yourself as a tree, with roots growing down into the earth through the soles of your feet. The energy of your being roots deep into the earth, and any excess energy is grounded within your strong roots. When you feel you are sufficiently anchored or earthed, bring yourself back into the room. Other grounding techniques include tai chi breathing, physical exercise, eating something, being in nature, and putting your hands into sand, soil, or running water.

Protecting Yourself

Whenever we are consciously working with our chakras, we open ourselves to receiving the universal healing energy and are more sensitive to the energies around us. To protect against draining energies, there are a number of techniques you can use.

A protection exercise

Wrap a protective cloak of light and vitality around yourself, covering from head to toe. Visualize it as any color that offers strength, comfort, and reassurance (I use lavender). Request that universal energy, God, or Goddess protect you from all negative energy.

Cleansing Yourself

Our chakras need cleansing regularly to get rid of unwanted energies absorbed from people, places, or situations. If you are feeling tired, drained, or emotionally unstable, you may be absorbing and carrying external energies, and this may have an influence on you. Daily cleansing will help to clear these energies and improve the circulation of your own energies.

It is also important to make sure that you have carried out a cleansing exercise before you self-heal. The clearer your chakras and aura are, the more healing energy you will be able to create, attract, and absorb. Flower essences and homeopathy are great for cleansing your energy field.

A cleansing exercise

First ground and protect yourself. Smudge sticks are a traditional way of cleansing, using a bound stick of sage and sweetgrass. Light the smudge stick and wave it around your body to cleanse your physical body, your aura, and chakras. If you have asthma or allergies, you might like to use a flower essence spray instead. Now start to get a sense of your auric energy field. Feel how far it extends out into the space around you. See and sense its layers with your inner vision. Ask the divine to remove all negative energy within your energy field immediately and to send it instantly to the Light. Ask the divine to cleanse, heal, and protect your energy field for the highest good. Once this cleansing exercise is complete, bring your focus back to your breathing and your physical body.

> **WISE WOMAN WAYS**
> All this grounding, protecting, and cleansing can sound a tad woolly; however, an awareness of your subtle energy and a willingness to engage with it in a practical way will help you feel calmer and more positive. I can't guarantee that, of course! But try it and see for yourself.

Using Healing for Yourself

To engage with chakra healing is simple. Find a quiet place, free from distraction. You may be sitting or lying down. Your eyes may be open or closed. Closed might encourage you to focus on your inner experience more. Take a few deep, slow breaths and relax your body as much as possible. Ground yourself and set your protection. Place your hand on the chakra and feel the warmth of your touch. Breathe into the place where your hand is—in and out, slowly and deeply. As you inhale, visualize breathing in peaceful, healing energy, and as you exhale, imagine this same energy flowing out of your hand and into the chakra.

Working With the Chakras
During the Menstrual Years

CHAKRA	1
Yin and Yang poles	Yin (receptive and feminine)
Location	Base of spine between anus and genitals at the perineum, connected to coccyx and opening downwards
Sensory function	Smell
Associated body parts	Skeletal system, adrenal glands, kidneys, anus, prostate, bladder, and genitals
Physical dysfunction	Osteoporosis and adrenal fatigue
Life issues	Survival, physical needs, standing up for oneself, physical health and fitness, grounding, stability, security, group power, and identity
Emotional dysfunction	Mental lethargy, "spaciness," victim mentality, unfocused mind, and distrust
Behavioral dysfunction	Difficulty achieving goals, over-activity, passivity, not looking after one's body
Color	Red/black

Element	Earth
Aromatherapy oils	Sandalwood, patchouli, and musk
Australian Bush Essences	Waratah, red lily (disconnection), sundew (indecisive), fringe violet (aura damage), grey spider (panic), macrocarpa (exhaustion), and bush iris (clearing blocks of physical excess and materialism)
Bach Flower Remedies	Rock rose (extreme panic and fears), clematis (daydreamer, too much time in the spirit realm, ungrounded), hornbeam (mental exhaustion), and aspen (vague fears of the unknown)
Quartz crystals	Red tiger's eye, garnet, red jasper, ruby, obsidian, hematite, agate, bloodstone, garnet, red coral, ruby, hematite, onyx, rose quartz, and smoky quartz
Yoga positions	Bridge, half and full locust, spinal roll, balancing, and child pose

Reflections

• What are your physical needs at this point in time?

I recognize when this chakra is out because I can get lower back pain and constipation, while psychologically I know that I'm not trusting myself or another person about something. If you excuse the pun, this chakra for me can be a pain the bum!

CHAKRA	2
Yin and Yang poles	Yang (positive and masculine)
Location	Lower abdomen, between naval and genitals, just above the anus, opens forward
Sensory function	Taste
Associated body parts	Circulatory system, uterus, ovaries, and testes glands
Physical dysfunction	Impotence, frigidity, bladder and prostate trouble, lower back pain, and erratic libido
Life issues	Emotional balance, sexuality, uncovering motivations, influencing choices based on conditioning, allowing pleasure, creative expression, partnerships, and playfulness
Emotional dysfunction	Instability, sadness, feelings of isolation, and martyr mentality
Behavioral dysfunction	Excessive libido and sexual withdrawal
Color	Orange
Element	Water
Aromatherapy oils	Melissa, orange, mandarin, neroli, sandalwood, and ylang ylang
Australian Bush Essences	Turkey bush (creativity), billy goat plum (releases shame), spinifex (cleansing, victim archetype), she oak (hormonal imbalance), and flannel flower (lack of sensitivity and sexual abuse)

Bach Flower Remedies	Agrimony, centaury, pine, larch, and gorse
Quartz crystals	Coral, carnelian, citrine, and golden topaz
Yoga positions	Cobra, pelvic rock, goddess pose, leg lifts, pelvic side rolls, downward facing dog, open legs, and hip circles

Reflections

- What influences might you be carrying from your past that influences your thoughts now?
- How are you allowing pleasure to enter your life?

Ah, the chakra of creative self-expression. At the time of writing this book, when my uterus has a fluid life of its own—my creative side is struggling to be birthed on a more profound level. I've never birthed a physical baby, but by jingo, birthing the baby of creativity surely comes a close second! The lesson of the sacral chakra is letting go of fear, anger, and controling behavior, so the purpose of the Sacred is achieved through emotional connections.

CHAKRA	3
Yin and Yang poles	Yin (receptive and feminine)
Location	Between naval and base of sternum, opens forward
Sensory function	Sight
Associated body parts	Digestive system, gallbladder, spleen, pancreas, and liver, limbic system, and adrenal glands

Physical dysfunction	Stomach ulcers, fatigue, weight around stomach, allergies, and diabetes
Life issues	Personal power, will, self-esteem/self-confidence, the courage to take risks, to be, purpose, effectiveness, endurance, self-respect, uniqueness, and individuality
Emotional dysfunction	Oversensitive to criticism, low self-esteem
Behavioral dysfunction	Aggressive, controlling, and addictions
Color	Yellow
Element	Fire
Aromatherapy oils	Rosemary, lemon, grapefruit, bergamot, ginger, ylang ylang, and cinnamon
Australian Bush Essences	Dynamis essence (combination of essences for energy), old man banksia (counteracts weariness), macrocarpa (energy), crowea (releases worry), wild potato bush (releases feeling physically encumbered), banksia robur (lethargy), bottlebrush (letting go), peach flowered tea tree, waratah, and five corners
Bach Flower Remedies	Cerato (strength to trust one's own judgment), larch (lack of self-confidence), schleranthus (indecisiveness), chicory, larch,

	pine, crab apple, and walnut
Quartz crystals	Citrine, amber, tigers eye, and yellow topaz
Yoga positions	Bow, pike pose, belly push, boat pose, front stretch, and warrior

Reflections

• Are you taking on too much responsibility? Do you need to delegate?

> **WISE WOMAN WAYS**
>
> Continue to develop a conscious awareness of your energetic anatomy. Sometimes I can be doing something inane and I become aware that my hand chakras are generating enormous heat. Waste not, want not—I channel this active healing energy to those in need.

CHAKRA	4
Yin and Yang poles	Yang (positive and masculine)
Location	Center of chest (breastbone), opens forward
Sensory function	Feeling
Associated body parts	Heart, chest, lungs, circulation, and thymus gland
Physical dysfunction	Shallow breathing, high blood pressure, heart disease, and cancer
Life issues	Beliefs about love and relationships, forgiveness and compassion for oneself and others, balance,

	compassion, self-acceptance, and unconditional acceptance of others
Emotional dysfunction	Co-dependency, melancholia; fears concerning loneliness, commitment, and/or betrayal
Behavioral dysfunction	Passivity and withdrawal
Color	Green/pink
Element	Air
Aromatherapy oils	Eucalyptus, pine, tea tree, bergamot, and melissa
Australian Bush Essences	Bush fuchsia (speaking your true essence), crowea (worry), turkey bush (creativity), red grevillia (becoming unstuck), flannel flower (intimacy), illawara flame tree (fear of rejection), sturt desert pea (emotional pain), bluebell, rough bluebell, and waratah
Bach Flower Remedies	Holly (blocked love), gorse (despair), and chicory
Quartz crystals	Aventurine, emerald, jade, malachite, peridot, rose quartz, watermelon tourmaline, green calcite, azurite, and moonstone
Yoga positions	Cobra, the fish, cow-face, breathing techniques

Reflections

- Are there some issues you feel ready to forgive others (or yourself) for?

This heart chakra is, for me, maybe the most poignant of all. To experience self-love and self-respect is most challenging. Yet how can we truly love another, or accept love from another, if we don't have this love and respect for the self?

CHAKRA	5
Yin and Yang poles	Yin (receptive and feminine)
Location	Centrally at base of neck, opens forward
Sensory function	Hearing
Associated body parts	Throat, ears, nose, teeth, mouth, neck, thyroid, and parathyroid glands
Physical dysfunction	Sore throats, neck ache, thyroid problems, hearing problems, tinnitus, and asthma
Life issues	Communication, self-expression, the power of choice, personal expression, harmony with others, self-knowledge, creativity
Emotional dysfunction	Perfectionism, inability to express emotions, and blocked creativity
Behavioral dysfunction	Withdrawal, people pleasing
Color	Light blue
Element	Sound
Aromatherapy oils	Geranium or bergamot
Bach Flower Remedies	Agrimony
Australian Bush Essences	Cognis essence (clarity and courage to speak truth, great for study and new information), paw paw

	(assimilating new information), turkey bush (creative blocks), old man banksia, flannel flower, bush fuchsia, mint bush
Quartz crystals	Sodalite, lapis lazuli, blue agate, aquamarine, turquoise, celestite, sapphire
Yoga positions	Neck rolls, shoulder stand, fish pose, the plough

Reflections

- To what extent are you able to free yourself from harmful external values and beliefs?
- To what extent are you able to express yourself and your beliefs?

Many years ago in my late twenties, I went through a particular growth phase when I was making connections with my "little Laurel" side and realizing how much of my inappropriate adult drives were happening because of unhealthy childhood conditioning. In one vision quest, I saw myself as a thin, naked little girl with a paper bag over her head. In the two weeks following this, I developed a cold and a horrendous cough, during which time (I hope this isn't too much information for you) phlegm caught in my throat by the bucketful necessitating an emergency visit by the doctor. My cough and cold came and went. More importantly, I learnt to express my feelings as an adult and to heal from past trauma.

CHAKRA	6
Yin and Yang poles	Yang (receptive and masculine)
Location	Above and between eyebrows, space behind forehead, opens forward
Sensory function	Sixth sense

Associated body parts	Eyes, base of skull, nose, ears, and pituitary gland
Physical dysfunction	Headaches, poor vision, neurological disturbances, glaucoma, and nightmares
Life issues	Intuition, wisdom, emotional intelligence, ability to "see" other than with the eyes
Emotional dysfunction	Seasonally depressed
Behavioral dysfunction	Learning difficulties and hallucinations
Color	Indigo
Element	Light
Aromatherapy oils	Patchouli, frankincense, and bergamot
Australian Bush Essences	Bush iris (clears blocks relating to grounding and trust), bush fuchsia (intuition), isopogon (memory), green spider orchid, and boronia
Bach Flower Remedies	Walnut, crab apple, rock water, and vervain
Quartz crystals	Tourmaline, tanzanite, lapis lazuli, sapphire, amethyst, purple apatite, azurite, calcite, and fluorite
Yoga positions	Palming, seated yoga mudra visualization and imagery

Reflections

- To what extent has your intuitive abilities sharpened?
- How do you balance your imagination and fantasy realm with reality?

- To what extent do you hide your intuition behind a rational mind?

CHAKRA	7
Yin and Yang poles	Yin and Yang
Location	Top/crown of head, position of fontanels, opens upward
Sensory function	None
Associated body parts	Upper skull, cerebral cortex, skin, pineal gland
Physical dysfunction	Sensitivity to pollution, chronic exhaustion, epilepsy, and Alzheimer's disease
Life issues	Spirituality, selflessness, expanded consciousness
Emotional dysfunction	Depression, obsessional thinking, confusion
Behavioral dysfunction	Obsessive-compulsive disorder (OCD)
Color	Violet, white, and gold
Element	Thought, cosmic energy
Aromatherapy oils	Frankincense
Australian Bush Essences	Red lily (disconnection), sundew (indecision), angelsword, bush iris, and waratah
Bach Flower Remedies	Wild oat (reconnecting)
Quartz crystals	Amethyst, diamond, clear quartz, white jade, white tourmaline, snowy quartz, and herkimer
Yoga positions	Headstand, seated meditation

Reflections

- To what extent do you experience the connection to the divine?
- To what extent do you experience unconditional love in other intimate relationships?

WISE WOMAN WAYS

RITUAL FOR AURA CLEANSING

Do the following exercise, before going to bed at night or if you have been exposed to negative or scattered energy:

Using the third and fourth fingers of both hands, press firmly on the point between the eyebrows. From there, with the same fingers, trace a line over the crown of the head and down to the back of the neck and then down the spine as far as you can reach.

Still using the same fingers, reach under your arms and around to the centre of your back to pick up at the point you left off in step 1 and continue, pressing firmly down the centre of the back, the backs of the legs (simultaneously) to the calves. Finish with a flick of the fingers.

With the third and fourth fingers of the right hand, start again at the point between the eyebrows and trace a line up and over the crown, down the back of the neck, back under your right side of your chin, and along the left shoulder and the front of the left arm. Finish the movement with a sharp flick.

Repeat the above, this time using the third and fourth fingers of the left hand and tracing the line over the head and down the front of the right arm. Using both hands, trace the line up from the point between the eyebrows over the head to the back of the neck.

Here the hands separate, down each side of the neck under the jaw line, over the front of the throat, to join again at the breastbone. In one continuous flowing movement and maintaining firm pressure, follow the center line down the front of the body with both hands and then (simultaneously), down both legs, finishing at the ankles, once again with a flick.

MENSTRUFACT

Ancient Egyptians used softened papyrus as rudimentary tampons. Hippocrates notes that the Greeks used lint wrapped around wood. The modern tampon was invented by Dr. Earle Haas in 1929, which was called a "catamenial device" or "monthly device." Dr. Haas trademarked the brand name Tampax.

What Happens Next?

Chakra healing can bring profundity into your life. Quartz crystal healing can further enhance this link. Let me tell you more.

CHAPTER 9

Quartz Crystal Healing
for Menstruation

The earth is composed of one-third quartz crystal, making it one of the most abundant compounds found on its surface and within most sedimentary, metamorphic, and igneous rocks. Quartz has also been found in lunar rocks. Did you know that:

- the silica and water that crystals are composed of are also major components of the physical body?
- quartz is fossilized water, and our bodies are 65–75 percent water?
- the piezoelectric effects of crystals (their energy fields) match the earth's magnetic field and the magnetic field of the human aura?

There is a huge variety of quartz and quartz derivatives, including the following: agate, amethyst, ametrine, aqua aura quartz, aventurine, black quartz, bloodstone, blue siberian quartz, candle quartz, carnelian, cathedral quartz, chalcedony, chrysoprase, citrine, clear quartz, drusy quartz, elestial quartz, faden quartz, fairy quartz, golden healer quartz, green Siberian quartz, heliotrope, jasper, lavender quartz, lepidocrosite herkimer, metamorphosis quartz, onyx, opal, phantom quartz, rock crystal, rose quartz, ruby aura quartz, rutilated quartz, sardonyx, smoky quartz, snow quartz, spirit quartz, starseed quartz, quartz, tigers eye, and tourmaline.

You can find quartz in many everyday items, including sandpaper, soap, ceramics, radios, and TVs. Quartz crystals were used in the first radio wave transceivers and were essential in the development of computers.

They are also used in watches and timepieces. When a crystal is put in a watch, the battery sends a constant charge through the crystal. The crystal absorbs the charge, then releases it at such a precise rate the watch is able to keep perfect time.

How Crystal Healing Works

The ancient Egyptians used lapis lazuli, turquoise, carnelian, emerald, and clear quartz in their jewelry and grave amulets. Stones were used for protection and health. A hieroglyphic papyrus from the year 2,000 BC documents a medical cure using crystal, and several papyruses from the year 1,500 BC documents additional cures.

Jade was seen as the concentrated essence of love and was recognized as a kidney healing stone both in China and South America. The original settlers of North, Central, and South America used crystals widely for spiritual, ceremonial, and healing purposes. Mayan Indians used quartz crystals for both the diagnosis and treatment of disease.

In Europe, from the 11th century through the Renaissance, a number of medical treatises appeared (Hildegard von Bingen, Arnoldus Saxo, and John Mandeville), extolling the virtues of precious and semiprecious stones in the treatment of ailments, alongside herbal remedies. The solar temple at Newgrange in the Boyne Valley of Ireland is older than the pyramids and was built so that the sun would stream through the 70-foot-long entrance tunnel on the Winter Solstice. Its roof was originally covered with white quartz[17] to symbolize the White Goddess.

Quartz crystals focus, structure, amplify, transmit, transform, and store energy because they:

- have an energy grid of their own that evolves;
- absorb the energy of the earth, nature, environment, events, and people around them and reveal their layers in response to different energies;

- have layers of growth and experience, as we do; and
- have their own karmic cycles.

American research scientist Marcel Vogel (1917–1991)[18] worked for IBM for 27 years and developed the magnetic coating for IBM's disc drive and the first liquid crystal displays (LCD). He believed that the inner structure of crystals are in a perfect state of balance and radiate energy in a coherent manner that could be used to heal negative thought forms at the base of disease. Marcel also designed the Vogel crystal, which focuses the universal life force.

Crystals affect our energetic anatomy (chakras and aura) fields, which surround and permeate the physical body. A quartz crystal may be held in the hand or placed around the body. The power of the crystal is directed to the part of the physical body or energetic anatomy that requires healing. Crystals complement other healing modalities. When placed on or around the body during a healing session, and used in conjunction with other healing modalities, such as shamanic healing or Reiki, the crystals work both independently and cooperatively on healing.

Crystals may be worn, placed in an environment (outside or inside), or even used in a distance healing capacity.

WISE WOMAN WAYS

I've always felt crystals, flowers, plants, herbs, and wood need to be placed together and try to do this aesthetically in the home as part of the décor.

Cleansing Crystals

Cleansing is the process of removing any previous energies and influences that a crystal may have either absorbed or come into contact with, whether during its production, handling, or environment of origin. It is a good idea to cleanse the crystals you work with on a regular basis.

Water

Place the crystal in a clear glass bowl filled with water. CAUTION: Some crystals are water-soluble, which means they can dissolve in water. Most water-soluble crystals end in "ite."

Salt

Most members of the quartz family are safe with salt, but some are not. Dissolve one teaspoon of natural sea salt in one pint of water and place your crystal in the water overnight. Make sure you rinse all traces of salt away from the crystal and allow the crystal to dry naturally. Or you can bury your crystal in a bowl of natural sea salt for eight hours. Make sure you brush away all remains of salt.

Smudging

You can smudge crystals with sage, myrrh, sandalwood, frankincense, lavender, cedar, thyme, rosemary, or sweetgrass to cleanse them. Either fan the incense over the crystals with a feather or pass the crystal through the smoke of burning herbs, incense, or essential oil several times.

Other crystals

You can cleanse your crystal by placing it on a large crystal cluster for several hours. Quartz clusters are self-cleaning and charging. Citrine is also a cleansing crystal in its own right.

Sunlight

You can cleanse your crystals by placing in direct sunlight (inside or outside), which is said to represent male energies. CAUTION: The sun will fade many crystals, including amethyst. Direct hot sun beaming through clear quartz may also be a fire hazard.

Moonlight

The moon can also cleanse crystals and is said to represent female energies. During the full moon, the moon's energy is enhanced and is a good time for cleaning crystals. Place the crystals outside or inside. CAUTION: Be aware of rain, if placing crystals outside. I've cleansed crystals this way many times and find it a wonderful experience. We have a very long, terraced garden, which slopes away from the house. Sometimes I've placed the crystals out at dusk, so I don't break my neck getting down the garden at night. I have placed extra protection around the crystal layout, and not once have I found any crystal missing or out of place the next morning (no matter what the fairies and foxes may do at night!).

Intent

Hold your crystal in your hands and imagine a golden light from above coming down and filling the crystal and cleansing it of all negativity.

Sound

All crystals love sound, and you can use a tuning fork, singing bowl, or Tibetan cymbals to cleanse your crystals. Use your choice of sound by playing the sound over and around your crystal. This is a useful technique for large crystals. You might place one crystal inside a singing bowl.

Reiki

If you are attuned to Reiki you can use it to cleanse your crystals. This can be done by placing the crystals in your hands or holding your hands over the crystal and asking the Reiki to flow to cleanse the crystal. This is also a handy technique for any large or awkward crystals.

WISE WOMAN WAYS

CRYSTAL CAVE MEDITATION

Sit or lie comfortably. Close your eyes. Relax your body and slow your breathing. Imagine walking up a woodland path in the spring sunshine. As you walk, the path becomes progressively steeper. As you come to the crest of the hill, you see an opening to your left, leading to a cave in the side of the hill, partially hidden by flowering bushes. Walk into the cave. The air is cool and you see a sparkle where the walls are covered with black opals and red carnelian, giving off a scarlet glow. Walk through the cave of rich red crystals, absorbing their light. You move into another cave. Slowly, the opals and carnelian give way to tangerine quartz glowing a vibrant orange. Walk through the tangerine quartz, absorbing their light. You're moving deeper down into the earth and into another cave. Slowly, the tangerine quartz gives way to citrine and golden tiger's eye, shining with a sunshiny yellow. Walk through the citrine and golden tiger's eye, absorbing their light. The citrine and golden tiger's eye give way to a cave of rose quartz and rainforest jasper. Walk through the crystals, absorbing their light. The crystals give way to a cave of turquoise crystals. Walk through the turquoise, absorbing its light. The turquoise gives way to walls of blue tiger's eye. Walk through the crystal cave, absorbing their light. Farther down and deeper you go.

The crystals give way to an amethyst cave. Walk through the amethyst, absorbing its light. Finally, you walk into the innermost cavern, which is completely covered in pure rock crystal. Sit for a while in harmony with the healing crystals and the quiet stillness of the earth before returning to the outer world.

Charging Crystals

You will need to recharge your crystals immediately after cleaning them. While your crystal already contains its own unique vibrational energies, those energies can sometimes become low or depleted. When you recharge crystals, you're basically giving them the chance to refresh their ability to focus and expand their energy.

Crystal clusters

Crystal cluster chunks, or caves, are known to be self-charging and will charge other crystals lain upon them.

Sound

Put a crystal near a single-note chime and strike the chime gently several times. This has a harmonizing effect on the crystal. If you like to chant, do so in the presence of your crystals. Put your crystal near a bell and gently produce a sound in it. Instead of using a bell you can use a resonant (tune) fork.

Reiki charging

If you are a Reiki I practitioner, you can charge your crystals with Reiki energy.

Sunlight

The ultraviolet light from the sun containing the full spectrum of light restores a crystal's energy. CAUTION: The sun will fade many crystals, such as amethyst. Direct hot sun beaming through clear quartz may also be a fire hazard.

Moonlight

Crystals can be recharged using the softened solar radiation reflected via the moon. CAUTION: Be aware of rain if placing outside.

> **WISE WOMAN WAYS**
>
> I have to confess to occasionally needing to cleanse and charge my crystals with not a lot of time to spare. As long as your intent is honorable and clear, it's wonderful how quickly the crystals will oblige! The crystals I have the privilege of working with may be used for teaching or healing. I offer a prayer for protection and of intent, asking that the crystals be cleansed of all negative energy and charged with the blessings of the Goddess for the highest good of all. I then smudge the room and the crystals.

Chakra Balancing With Crystals

One of the simplest ways to use crystals is as a means of balancing the chakra system. To realign chakra energies, place one or two crystals of the appropriate color on each chakra area for a few minutes.

First (root or base) chakra

How it can help: This will balance physical energy, motivation, and practicality and promote a sense of reality. It's a good idea to place a grounding stone like smoky quartz or black tourmaline between the feet to act as an anchor.

Related quartz crystals: Red tourmaline, onyx, red aventurine, red carnelian, red chalcedony, red-brown agate, ruby aura quartz, rutilated quartz, black smoky quartz, grey banded and Botswana agate, rainbow jasper, red and brecciated jasper, and red tiger's eye.

Second (sacral or spleen) chakra

How it can help: May help balance creativity and release blocks in your life that prevent pleasure.

Related quartz crystals: Carnelian, carnelian agate, drusy quartz, fire agate, fire opal, lepidocrosite included in quartz or amethyst, orange phantom quartz, Oregon opal, red jasper, and chryoprase.

Third (solar plexus) chakra

How it can help: To reduce anxiety, clear thoughts, and improve confidence.

Related quartz crystals: Citrine, spirit quartz, lemon chryoprase, opal aura quartz, smoky citrine, sunshine aura quartz, yellow jasper, yellow phantom quartz, yellow tourmaline, sculpture in quartz, golden healer quartz, rutilated quartz, and golden tiger's eye.

Fourth (heart) chakra

How it can help: To promote a sense of calm, create a sense of direction in life, and balance your relationship with others and the world. A pink stone can be added for emotional clearing.

Related quartz crystals: Aventurine, apple aura quartz, chryoprase, dentric agate, green agate, green aventurine, green jasper, helitrope, leopardskin jasper (jaguar stone), moss agate, olive jasper, peach aventurine, pink agate, pink carnelian, pink chalcedony, pink tourmaline, rainforest jasper, rose aura quartz, smoky rose quartz, strawberry quartz, green tourmaline, and rose quartz.

Fifth (throat) chakra

How it can help: To bring peace, ease communication difficulties, and promote self-expression.

Related quartz crystals: Aqua aura, blue aventurine, blue chalcedony, blue jasper, blue lace agate, blue phantom quartz, blue tiger's eye, blue-green agate, moss agate, tourmaline, water opal (hyalite), watermelon tourmaline, avalonite (drusy blue chalcedony), and blue agate.

Sixth (brow) chakra

How it can help: To promote intuitive skills and memory and increase understanding and self-knowledge.

Related quartz crystals: Amethyst, blue jasper, blue tiger's eye, chrysophal (blue-green opal) smoky quartz, and moss agate.

Seventh (crown) chakra

How it can help: This will integrate and balance all aspects of the self—physical, mental, emotional, and spiritual—and will promote positive thought patterns, inspiration, and imagination.

Related quartz crystals: Amethyst, amethyst spirit quartz, Botswana agate, lavender quartz, lavender amethyst, rock crystal, moonstone, ametrine, and clear quartz.

Crystals for Different Menstrual States

Pregnancy State	Quartz Crystal
Apprehension, anxiety, worry	Amethyst, aventurine, clear quartz, rose quartz, smoky quartz, black tourmaline, blue lace agate, watermelon tourmaline, carnelian, green aventurine, Herkimer diamond, Siberian quartz, jasper, fire agate,

smoky quartz, and jasper (chakras: brow, heart, solar plexus)

Constipation
Smoky quartz, black tourmaline, red jasper, and citrine

Depression
Amethyst, elestial quartz, smoky quartz, rose quartz, carnelian, amethyst, smoky quartz, black tourmaline, rutilated quartz, lithium quartz, ametrine, Botswana agate, carnelian, moss agate, tiger's eye, purple tourmaline, and Siberian quartz (chakra: solar plexus)

Fatigue
Clear quartz, yellow jasper, black tourmaline, Peru opal, amethyst, rose quartz, carnelian, fire agate, ametrine, blue opal, dendritic agate (chakra: base), fire opal, and rutilated quartz

Fuzzy thinking
Clear quartz, black tourmaline, amethyst, smoky quartz, opal, moss agate, green tourmaline, and red jasper (chakras: brow, crown)

Indecisive, self-doubting
Carnelian, smoky quartz, and tiger's eye

Insomnia
Amethyst, smoky quartz, candle quartz, moonstone, chrysoprase, and rose quartz (chakra: brow)

Intolerant, critical, irritable
Rose quartz

Low self-esteem
Rose quartz, moss agate, and chrysoberyl, citrine, opal, tourmaline (chakras: base, spleen, heart)

Lack of sexual interest	Carnelian, rose quartz (chakra: brow, base)
Panic	Green tourmaline
Backache	Green tourmaline and blue agate
Nausea or sickness	Moonstone and red jasper
Headache	Rose quartz, amethyst, blue lace agate, citrine, and moonstone
Water retention	Moonstone
Cramps	Moonstone, carnelian, rose quartz, amethyst, and citrine
To regulate cycle	Red jasper, bloodstone, moonstone, and carnelian

> **WISE WOMAN WAYS**
>
> Massaging with crystals combines the relaxing benefits of massage with the healing energy of crystals. If feeling stressed or headachy choose smooth clear quartz crystals such as spheres (I use the smooth end of a wand, one for either side of the head), tumble stones, or palm stones. Circle the crystal gently around the temples and over the forehead.

Ways to Use Crystals

In grids

A crystal grid involves using six single-pointed crystals (I would suggest using clear quartz or amethyst). If you are laying down, place one by your left foot with the point going up, one by your elbow, point up, and one by the left of your head point up. Then place one by the right of your head point going down, one by your elbow, point down, and one by your right foot, point down.

If you are sitting in a chair, place a crystal by your left foot going up, one just behind the chair on your left going up, one just behind the chair on your right going down, and one by your right foot, going down. You may choose to hold a crystal in your hand.

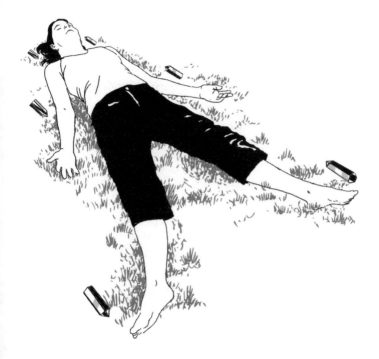

Gem essences

Gem essences can be dropped under the tongue, rubbed into pulse or chakra points, sprayed into the aura, put in bath water, or sprayed around a room. The basic principle behind the use of gem essences is the same as that of flower essences, in that when crystals are activated by natural sunlight or moonlight, they transfer their vibrational signature into water, creating a remedy that is safe and can be used in conjunction with all healing modalities. Once you have your gem essence, you can enhance it with flower essences. Put two drops of the chosen flower essences into the gem mixture. This is a particularly nice way to blend the energies of Bach Flower Remedies or Australian Bush Flower Essences with crystals. NOTE: Some crystals are toxic if taken internally.

Other Ways to Use Crystals

You could wear crystals on a waist chain, on acupressure points on the ear, on a bracelet or chain between your breasts, place it under your pillow, or hold it while meditating. Experiment with placing crystals at strategic points in a room.

> **WISE WOMAN WAYS**
> Make up a crystal power pouch containing the crystals of your choice, plus some sage for cleansing negativity, and carry it with you.

> **MENSTRUFACT**
> Studies suggest that city lights or artificial lights influence the menstrual cycle.

What Happens Next?

Crystals are a gift to you from Mother Earth and can be used as part of your energy healing during your menstrual cycle. Another Wise Woman healing art that uses energy healing is hand reflexology, which you can easily learn and do anywhere to help comfort and soothe any distress. Interested to know more? Read on…

CHAPTER 10

Hand Reflexology
for Menstruation

Whilst the art of reflexology dates back to Ancient Egypt, India, and China, it wasn't until 1913 that Dr. William Fitzgerald[19] introduced this therapy to the West as Zone Therapy. Dr. Fitzgerald researched how reflex areas on the feet and hands were linked to areas and organs of the body within the same zone. During the 1930s, Eunice Ingham[20] further developed this zone theory into what is now known as reflexology, observing that congestion in any part of the foot was mirrored in the corresponding part of the body.

What Is Hand Reflexology?

The feet are rich in nerve endings, which are why they are traditionally used by reflexologists to stimulate the flow of energy throughout the body, but the hands (and other key areas of the body) can also be used successfully, as discussed below. Hand reflexology can be self-administered anywhere and can bring ease and comfort during menstruation.

Hand reflexology contraindications

The main hand reflexology contraindications are as follows:

- Don't do it on broken skin or if there are infected sores or lesions on the hands
- Don't do hand reflexology if you have a hand injury.
- If you have any medical problem, consult a doctor first.

If you can't use your fingers or knuckles, use the blunt end of a pencil or the blunt end of a crystal wand.

Hand reflexology techniques

You may use all these techniques in one session, or just one technique:

1. RUBBING: Briskly rubbing your palms together will generate energy (chi) in them. Rubbing is also part of the hand reflexology routine.

2. SQUEEZING: Using your thumb pad and index finger to firmly squeeze each finger and thumb on the other hand, from base to tip.

3. PULLING: Using your thumb pad and index finger to firmly grasp the base of each finger and thumb on the other hand and pull down towards the tip.

4. PRESSING: Using the tip of your thumb to press and stimulate points on the opposite hand (you will need short nails!). Press until you feel pressure. Hold the pressure and work the point with rotary, or circular, pressure.

5. ROTARY, OR CIRCULAR PRESSURE: Press into the point and move in very small firm circles using a knuckle of the other hand or the blunt end of a pencil or crystal wand. I would recommend a rose quartz wand or maybe amethyst with a little essential oil on the blunt end (not too much or the wand will slip).

6. THUMB ROLL: Rolling the pad of your thumb over the points.

Massage the relevant points on both hands a couple of times a day. Hand pressure points adapt to stimulation, so after seven days stop for three days. If the symptoms persist, continue for another week (or more) or choose new points to press and work.

> **WISE WOMAN WAYS**
> You could put a flower essences mixture in the center of your palms before giving yourself hand reflexology. Or mix a little essential oil in with some hand cream and rub into your hands before giving yourself hand reflexology. Not too much, otherwise your fingers will skid everywhere!

Self-treatment

1. Begin your hand reflexology treatment by sitting quietly and closing your eyes. Take a few deep breaths as you still your body and focus your mind.
2. Pinch the tips of each finger of your left hand firmly (nail to back). Reverse and repeat this process on your right hand.
3. Go back to each fingertip and pinch them again, this time squeezing from side to side.
4. Vigorously rub from base to tip of each finger of your left hand, front and back plus sides. Reverse and repeat this process on your right hand.
5. Tug each finger and thumb firmly.
6. Using your right thumb and forefinger, grasp the webbed area between your thumb and forefinger of your left hand and tug gently. Repeat this process for the areas between all your fingers. Reverse and repeat on your right hand.
7. Turn your left hand palm down. Use your right thumb to massage the back of your hand, the knuckles and in-between area first, then all other areas. Reverse and repeat this process on your right hand.
8. Hold your left wrist (palm up) inside your right hand. Use your thumb to massage your inner wrist. Reverse and repeat this process on your right hand.

9. Massage the palm of your left hand with your right thumb, knuckle, or the blunt end of a crystal wand. Massage the fleshier mound areas more deeply. Reverse and repeat this process on your right hand.

10. At the end of the session press your right thumb or the blunt end of a crystal wand deeply in the center of your left palm. Reverse and repeat this process on your right hand. Take a few deep breaths and center yourself.

> **WISE WOMAN WAYS**
> If you are a Reiki II or III practitioner, activate your hand chakras before giving yourself hand reflexology.

Specific Menstruation Points

BACK PAIN: Work the spine points, which run along the outer edge of the thumb down towards the wrist. Apply rotary pressure along this area with the other hand. The point where the center of your hand joins your wrist can be stimulated to give relief from lower back pain.

BREAST TENDERNESS: Work the breast reflex on the left hand (top of hands under fingers) by rubbing using gentle but firm pressure using the thumb of the right hand. Reverse and repeat this process on your right hand.

FATIGUE: Work the adrenal reflex on the left hand with your right. Find the webbing between thumb and index finger and go into the palm about an inch. Apply a rotary pressure on the area indicated using the thumb or knuckle of the right hand. Reverse and repeat this process on your right hand. Do not work this reflex if you have high blood pressure.

HEADACHES: Apply rotary pressure all around the nail area of the left thumb with your other hand. Reverse and repeat on the right hand.

ANXIETY: Find the skin crease that runs right across your wrist at the base of your hand. The point is almost at the end of the crease, just inside the edge of the wrist bone (little finger side). Use your thumb pad to press the point until you feel a strong pressure. Hold the pressure while you knead the point using rotary movements for about 1 minute. Repeat on the other wrist. Press both points 2–3 times a day or whenever you feel anxious.

The ears (like the feet and hands) contain reflexology points corresponding to major body parts and areas. Sit with your back straight. Use your thumbs and your index fingers to rub and gently pull your ears from the top to bottom. You can also use the tips of your index fingers to rub the inside surface of both ears. Start at the ear opening and work your way to the outside edge, rubbing all the curves and folds of each ear, including behind your ears. Do this for 1–2 minutes per ear.

NAUSEA OR SICKNESS: I'm using an acupressure tip for this one. With your left palm up, measure three fingers' width (using your right hand) down from the first crease where your wrist bends. Where your index finger falls, feel along the crease for a slight dip in the groove between the two large tendons. Apply pressure at that point with your thumb and index finger (both sides of the wrist) for 1–2 minutes. Repeat with your other hand.

CONSTIPATION: Massage the dip in the palms of both hands with a clockwise movement.

PERIOD PAIN: To alleviate period pain, locate the uterus reflexes, which are at the base of the thumb side of both hands. This is best done pre-period as it may increase blood flow during a period. Grasp your wrist with your thumb and finger and twist the wrist from side to side. In addition press and rotate in the small dip located on the wrist directly underneath.

Helpful Reflexology Points
for Menstruation

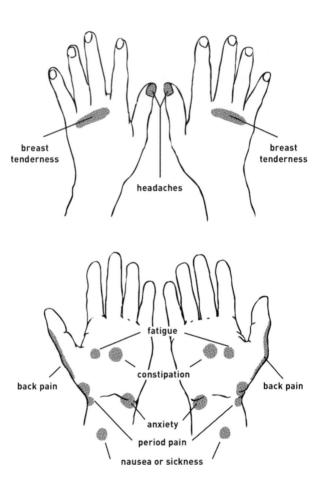

WISE WOMAN WAYS

Sometimes my lower back gets a little temperamental, especially just before my period, so I use hand reflexology to ease the discomfort. I tend to use my knuckles (especially the corner of a knuckle), and I use very small movements as I move down the spinal area on the thumbs.

MENSTRUFACT

In some parts of India, a woman indicates she is menstruating by wearing a handkerchief around her neck stained with her menstrual blood.

What Happens Next?

Let's move from the body-centered focus of the last few chapters to a place where you can create rituals to celebrate and honor the journey through your monthly cycle.

CHAPTER 11

Creating Rituals

Rituals provide us with a sense of security and stability—from plant-ing the spring bulbs to celebrating Yuletide. Ritual is different from habit. Habit, such as walking the dog, can be mindless but necessary, while ritual is an intentional, focused action. Ritual can create signifi-cance and celebration throughout the monthly cycle and offers opportu-nities to create harmony, patience, and appreciation in our lives. Rituals can be created for first blood (the first period) or to mark your evolving connection between your moontime and the Goddess.

Creating Sacred Space

Space is all around us. It can be full or empty. It can be literal (the kitchen) or abstract (our mind). Sacred can mean a special place to commune with yourself and the divine, whether it is God, Goddess, or something else. It is a space to be treated with reverence, set apart from the mundane. We can create a sacred space anywhere we choose—in-side a building or outside in nature. If we want to perform a ritual, alone or in company, we need to create sacred space.

> **WISE WOMAN WAYS**
>
> Stand naked in front of a mirror by candlelight and create your anointing oil by mixing extra-virgin olive oil with frank-incense or sandalwood. Ground and protect yourself and cast your sacred space. Take a drop of your mixture on your index finger and touch each chakra in turn while saying the following aloud:

- **CROWN:** Bless me, Goddess, that my spirit may be clear and true.
- **THIRD EYE:** Bless my inner vision, that I may see with insight.
- **THROAT:** Bless my self-expression, that I may speak with wisdom.
- **HEART:** Bless my heart, that it be open and filled with compassion.
- **SOLAR PLEXUS:** Bless my sense of self-esteem, that I may be true to myself.
- **SACRAL:** Bless my womb, that I may connect with the source of my creativity.
- **ROOT:** Bless my yoni, the gateway of life and death.
- **BOTTOMS OF FEET:** Bless my feet, that I may symbolically walk my path with courage.
- **PALMS OF HANDS:** Bless my hands, that I may symbolically give with unconditional love.

Casting Your Circle of Sacred Space

What we are doing when we cast a circle of sacred space is defining an area to be used for contemplation, meditation, or healing. This is the method I use when I am creating a sacred space. You can adapt it to suit your own needs:

1. Cleanse your area of work by, for example, smudging the area, use your besom (broom) to symbolically clear away negativity, or using "singing bowls" to clear the space.
2. Ground and protect yourself.
3. Have everything inside your circle that you are likely to need.
4. Stand facing outwards at the eastern point. Place your hands together at the heart chakra, and bring your hands up to a

point above your head as far as you can go. Say (silently or otherwise): "Guardian of the East and the element of Air, I call upon your presence and protection during this sacred healing." As you say the words, draw your hands apart in a wide circle until they meet palms and fingertips together at your second (sacral) chakra. Walk to the southern point.

5. Stand facing outwards at the southern point. Place your hands together at the heart chakra, and bring your hands up to a point above your head as far as you can go. Say (silently or otherwise): "Guardian of the South and the element of Fire, I call upon your presence and protection during this sacred healing." As you say the words, draw your hands apart in a wide circle until they meet palms and fingertips together at your second (sacral) chakra. Walk to the western point.

6. Stand facing outwards at the western point. Place your hands together at the heart chakra, and bring your hands up to a point above your head as far as you can go. Say (silently or otherwise): "Guardian of the West and the element of Water, I call upon your presence and protection during this sacred healing." As you say the words, draw your hands apart in a wide circle until they meet palms and fingertips together at your second (sacral) chakra. Walk to the northern point.

7. Stand facing outwards at the northern point. Place your hands together at the heart chakra, and bring your hands up to a point above your head as far as you can go. Say (silently or otherwise): "Guardian of the North and the element of Earth, Lord and Lady/God and Goddess, I call upon your presence and protection during this sacred healing." As you say the words, draw your hands apart in a wide circle until they meet palms and fingertips together at your second (spleen) chakra. Walk to the eastern point.

8. Stand facing inwards at the eastern point, and point from where you are with the index finger of your dominant hand or with a crystal wand. Trace a clockwise circle of protection around you (and the other person if appropriate) or altar. Visualize the circle strong and protective around you, going deep down into the Earth and upwards to the sky. Ask the God and Goddess (or your choice) that all within the circle come under the full protection of the God and Goddess at all times.

9. When the circle is complete with your energy, you should declare what the circle is for. A statement that this circle is created in love and compassion for self-healing, for example.

> **WISE WOMAN WAYS**
> I find a certain amount of comfort in ritual. Maybe, it's the familiarity and safety that allow creative energy to build. However, it's also true that stepping into the energetic abyss armed with good grounding and protection can invite a level of inspiration unavailable when dealing with the purely familiar.

Having cast your circle, you must always close it after your work is complete. This is the method I use. You can adapt it to suit your needs:

1. Stand facing outwards at the eastern point. Place your hands together at the heart chakra, and bring your hands up to a point above your head as far as you can go. Say (silently or otherwise): "Guardian of the East and the element of Air, I thank you for your presence and protection during this sacred healing. I bid you farewell." As you say the words,

draw your hands apart in a wide circle until they meet palms and fingertips together at your second (spleen) chakra. Walk to the southern point.

2. Stand facing outwards at the southern point. Place your hands together at the heart chakra, and bring your hands up to a point above your head as far as you can go. Say (silently or otherwise): "Guardian of the South and the element of Fire, I thank you for your presence and protection during this sacred healing. I bid you farewell." As you say the words, draw your hands apart in a wide circle until they meet palms and fingertips together at your second (spleen) chakra. Walk to the western point.

3. Stand facing outwards at the western point. Place your hands together at the heart chakra, and bring your hands up to a point above your head as far as you can go. Say (silently or otherwise): "Guardian of the West and the element of Water, I thank you for your presence and protection during this sacred healing. I bid you farewell." As you say the words, draw your hands apart in a wide circle until they meet palms and fingertips together at your second (spleen) chakra. Walk to the northern point.

4. Stand facing outwards at the northern point. Place your hands together at the fourth (heart) chakra, and bring your hands up to a point above your head as far as you can go. Say (silently or otherwise): "Guardian of the North and the element of Earth, God and Goddess (or your choice), I thank you for your presence and protection during this sacred healing. I bid you farewell." As you say the words, draw your hands apart in a wide circle until they meet palms and fingertips together at your second (spleen) chakra. Walk to the eastern point.

5.   Stand facing inwards at the eastern point, and point from where you are point with your dominant hand, palm down and fingers outstretched, or use a crystal wand. Trace a counter-clockwise circle around you and the other person or altar. Visualize the circle melting around you.

Although I have done many rituals in a modest way, I was nervous about casting my first circle. In fact, it was only after a dream where I was casting a circle, did I begin doing it for real. Even now, I am private in my rituals. A couple of years ago, I was doing a ritual alone in the garden, arms outstretched upwards—going great guns. I heard a noise behind me and saw my husband who had come home early from work, sitting quietly watching me. Although I know Mick has great respect for my beliefs, I still found it difficult when I knew he was watching.

WISE WOMAN WAYS

An altar helps set your focus for rituals, ceremonies, and healing. This space should be large enough for you to conduct your work upon. It might be a permanent table or a table you put up and take down for use anywhere. I have "spaces" rather than altars. For example, there are spaces in my healing room for crystals. On the nightstand next to my side of the bed is an amethyst crystal with some night-time Bach Rescue Remedy, plus a homeopathic remedy (all energy medicine). When the mood takes me, I put some flowers and greenery from the garden there as well, so the last thing I see at night is nature (or my lovely husband or maybe one of my four black cats peering down at me!).

You may choose to represent the four elements on your altar or sacred space with the following suggested articles:

- AIR: candles, feathers, smudge stick
- FIRE: candle, incense, a small cauldron, smudge stick, an oil burner, a vessel to burn herbs on
- WATER: floating candle, flowers in water, a ritual chalice with water in
- EARTH: plant, a small branch, crystals/gems, a vessel to burn herbs on

Before you begin any ritual, you should cleanse the area where the work is to be done and then cast the circle, as noted above. Once your work is complete, shut down the energy used for your workings, as discussed earlier, by thanking the guides, teachers, or God/Goddess that you called or who came into the circle to offer assistance. Then imagine the energy around the circle lowering around you fading. Finally, clear the space with a blessing and ask the energies to close the spiritual gateways.

First Blood

At the time when we have our first period, we are crossing the bridge from girlhood to womanhood. This rite of passage is a wonderful opportunity to mark an important event in a young girl's life.

Consider how it might have been if your mother and elder sisters, extended family, and friends had celebrated your first menstruation and welcomed you into womanhood. What if you were told how wonderful the gifts of menstruation were and its profundity explained to you. How might you have felt about being a woman? How might you have felt about your body and its functions? Would that celebration having affected how you feel now? If your experience was less than ideal, the following is a suggestion to inspire you with possible ways of rewriting your past.

Choose a quiet place and create your sacred space. Ground and protect yourself. Remember and write out your first blood experience, detailing the practicalities of being told (if you were) and your first period. Consider how you felt, physically and psychologically. It may be that you hold resentment against those who could have guided you better at that time. Picture them. Give your forgiveness to them as much as possible. Give yourself some time to allow this process to happen. When you are ready, picture yourself as you were then. Write out how you would tell yourself as a young girl about menstruation. Consider the advice and support you would give to yourself. Be kind and gentle. Be loving with yourself. Allow time to write and reflect. When you are ready, return to the present and move on.

WISE WOMAN WAYS

What was your first bleeding like? Joyful? Fearful? Happy? Shameful? What was the reaction of your parents, family, and friends to your first bleed? Was your first blood celebrated or ignored? When I worked on this chapter, I felt sad remembering how I entered my early period years. There was no space in my family to honor or support this sacred time. Although I have done much work on how I relate to my femininity and inner self over the years, and this has made my periods easier to manage, it is only now I realize how lonely the journey has been. For the women who are parents reading this book, I would ask you to consider your daughter's transition from girlhood to womanhood and how you may work with her to celebrate this time. She will carry the experience with her for the rest of her life and be the better for it.

Creating a ceremony

Do you want to create a ceremony for first blood or menstruation? Why do you want to mark it? If you would like to enable healing, what healing and why? It could be that you would like to state your beliefs and express your hope for the future. What beliefs? What are your hopes?

Preparing for the ceremony

Where would you like the ceremony? Who would you like to witness the ceremony? Do you want any special clothing?

Opening the ceremony

You might like to include candle lighting, music, essential oils or incense, a blessing, or a statement of intent.

Main body of the ceremony

You might like to include candle lighting, chanting, drumming, meditation, essential oils or incense, hand or foot washing, planting something, reading text, storytelling, exchanging or giving gifts, creating amulets, singing, music, dancing, prayers and blessings, immersion in water, anointing, guided meditation or visualization, silence, or the use of ritual objects.

Closing the ceremony

You could close with a blessing, music, or sharing of food and drink.

Marking Your Moontime
and Goddess Connection

"Moontime" is a term for menstruation that links a woman's monthly cycle to that of the moon's cycle. Across many cultures, the moon has symbolized renewal, the feminine, and eternity. As it waxes and wanes, the moon can be seen to control both the oceans and menstrual blood.

A woman's bleeding was considered a cosmic event, connecting the woman to the lunar cycles and tides. She was thought to be at the height of her power at this time, and for this reason was encouraged to listen to her inner voice, which would often bring forth wisdom of benefit to the tribe or community. In ancient times, over 25,000 years ago, calendars were found made out of bone that are believed to link the menstrual and moon cycles. The word "menstruation" comes from the Greek *menus,* meaning both "moon" and "power," and *men,* meaning "month."

In her book, *A Woman's Book of Life,* Joan Borysenko writes that the female body becomes attuned to the lunar energy cycles at puberty. Studies have shown that ovulation (and peak conception) occurs around the full moon. She suggests that women are more outgoing and creative when estrogen levels are high (just before ovulation) and more inner directed when progesterone levels are high (just before menstruation). During the new moon, ovulation and conception rates are shown to decrease overall, and more women start menstruating at this time. Progesterone and estrogen both decrease, and women's psychic abilities seem to be heightened.

Choose to do a moontime ritual on the first day of your cycle, outside or inside, day or night. Set up your altar with symbols that reflect the power of the creative feminine such as shells, water, flowers, moon-shaped objects, specific stones, candles (white for the Maiden aspect, red for the Mother aspect, and black for the Crone aspect). Call on whichever guides and Goddesses you feel close to (see Chapter 2). Ask them to aid you in your quest to balance your feminine energy. Say any specific prayers, sing, drum, or chant. Close the ritual and enjoy some food or drink. Write in your journal about your moods, health, energy levels, and dreams at the time.

WISE WOMAN WAYS

Create your own Moon Lodge. Set aside a room or corner for this time. Choose comfortable pillows and blankets in beautiful colors, flowers or plants, and incense or essential oils for burning. This is your sacred time for resting, rejuvenation, and meditation. Women tend to be very grounding to others during this time. You might choose to do healing work with other women who are menstruating, as sharing this work can lead to powerful results.

Suggested rituals for your moontime:

- CREATE A MOON CORD OF THIN RED CORD: Tie it around your waist under your clothes and wear it each day of your period, to remind yourself of the sacredness of this time.
- CREATE A BATH RITUAL: Prepare with candles, music, essential oils (adding after you have run the bath), crystals, and a glass of water or cup of herbal tea. As you lay in the bath, consider any issues in your life at the moment and choose one issue that you can creatively change and decide what you will do about it in the coming month. Secondly, offer your gratitude for the blessings in your life. Then just relax and enjoy the water until you're ready to get out.
- CREATE A SPECIAL TEA: Create a special tea blend that you drink during menstruation.
- READ AN INSPIRATIONAL BOOK ON WOMEN.
- MAKE A MENSTRUAL JOURNAL: Make a menstrual journal by covering a notebook with fabric or pasting pic-

tures on it that you like and use it to record your menstrual intuitions, inspirations, and dreams.

- FOCUS ON THE COLOR RED: Wear red lipstick. Paint your nails red. Henna your hair. Wear red underwear. Light red candles. Wear rubies, garnet, or moonstone.
- GO TO BED IN THE DAYTIME: Lay in bed all afternoon, just sleeping and dreaming.
- RECEIVE A HEALING SESSION: Schedule an appointment for a massage or other healing therapy at the end of your moontime.
- SPLASH YOUR BODY WITH ROSEWATER.

For more ideas, see *105 Ways to Celebrate Menstruation* by Kami McBride.

WISE WOMAN WAYS

In cultures of the past, a community of women, such as those living in a village, would almost all ovulate at the full moon and bleed at the dark moon. The ovulation moon is called the white moon cycle, and the outer (moon) and inner (the woman) energies match the power of the full moon, enhancing a woman's fertility and Mother Goddess energies. The bleed moon is called a red moon cycle, where the full moon lends its energy to a woman's menstruation, enhancing her inner development and Crone Goddess energies. Today, most women's cycles still fall into one or the other types, particularly if they attune to the moon. It is also quite common for close friends or work colleagues to have their periods at the same time.

Let's talk about making love during your moontime. Practically speaking, I suggest you wait until your heaviest bleed days have passed and cover the surface where you're having sex with a towel (keeping wet wipes within reach for a quick clean up). If you want to experiment with different positions but don't want the mess, insert a cervical cap, diaphragm, or menstrual cup (an alternative to tampons and pads—not a method of contraception) before intercourse. The best position for least mess is having your partner on top.

If you ovulate early, you can still get pregnant if you have unprotected sex during your period (sperm can survive inside a woman's body for up to seven days). Also be aware that having unprotected sex during your period could make you more prone to infections.

During my younger years, I often made love towards the end of my period. My hormones were more rampant, and patience was never one of my virtues. Many women have told me they feel more passionate and sexually wild during their bleed than at any other time in their cycle. So whatever floats your boat, ladies.... Enjoy!

Tantrism is an ancient yoga practice, which involves *maithuna*, sacred sexual intercourse, the purpose of which is spiritual enlightenment. The optimal time for this to occur is during a woman's bleed when her sexual energy is at its peak. In tantric sex, making love during a woman's moontime is special and intimate and the aftermath may offer a time of increased intuitive and visionary perceptions.

WISE WOMAN WAYS

In *Buffalo Woman Comes Singing*, Brooke Medicine Eagle writes that many of the modern prophecies made by Native peoples were made by women in their Moon Lodges.

MENSTRUFACT

The English word "taboo" comes from the Polynesian word *tapua*, meaning both "sacred" and "menstruation."

What Happens Next?

Your menstrual journey spans many years and offers pathways to self-discovery that are sacred and priceless. As a wise woman coming to the end of her menstrual journey and now entering the mysteries of menopause, I give you the gift that many women who have gone before have given to me: I give you yourself.

Further Reading

Aubyn, Lorna St. *Everyday Rituals and Ceremonies*. London, UK: Piatkus, 1998.

Baring, Anne and Jules Cashford. *The Myth of the Goddess: Evolution of an Image*. London, UK: Arkana Penguin, 1993.

Borysenko, Joan, *A Woman's Book of Life: The Biology, Psychology, and Spirituality of the Feminine Life Cycle.* New York, NY: Riverhead Books, 1988.

Capacchione, Lucia. *The Creative Journal*. Pompton Plains, NJ: New Page Books, 2002.

Conway D.J. *Maiden, Mother, Crone*. Woodbury, MN: Llewellyn Publications, 1994.

Crawford, C. *Daughters of the Inquisition.* Tensed, ID: Seven Springs Press, 2004.

Davis, Martha and Elizabeth Robbins Eshelman. *The Relaxation & Stress Reduction Workbook.* Oakland, CA: New Harbinger Publications, 2000.

Durdin-Robertson, L. *The Cult of the Goddess*. Enniscorthy, Eire: Cesara Publications, 1974.

Eden, Donna. *Energy Medicine*. London, UK: Piatkus, 2008.

Ewing, Jim Pathfinder. *Finding Sanctuary in Nature*. Forres, Scotland: Findhorn Press, 2007.

Farrar, Janet and Farrar, Stewart. *The Witches' Goddess: The Feminine Principle of Divinity*. London, UK: Robert Hale, 1987.

Francia, Luisa. *Dragontime: Magic and Mystery of Menstruation.* Woodstock, NY: Ash Tree Publishing, 1991.

Gienger, Michael. *Healing Crystals*. Forres, Scotland: Findhorn Press, 2005.

FURTHER READING

Gienger, Michael. *Crystal Massage for Health and Healing*. Forres, Scotland: Findhorn Press, 2006.

Gienger, Michael and Joachim Goebal. *Gem Water*. Forres, Scotland: Findhorn Press, 2008.

Gray, Linda. *Grow Your Own Pharmacy*. Forres, Scotland: Findhorn Press, 2007.

Guhr, Andreas and Jorg Nagler. *Crystal Power: Mythology and History*. Forres, Scotland: Findhorn Press, 2006.

Harvey, Clare. *The New Encyclopedia of Flower Remedies*. London, UK: Watkins Publishing, 2007.

Harvey, Graham. *Listening People, Speaking Earth: Contemporary Paganism* (Second Edition). London, UK: Hurst and Company, 2007.

Jacobson, E. *Progressive Relaxation*. Chicago, IL: University of Chicago Press, 1938.

Judith, Anodea and Slen Vega. *The Sevenfold Journey*. Freedom, CA: Crossing Press, 1993.

Keet, Michael and Louise. *Hand Reflexology: Stimulate Your Body's Healing System*. London, UK: Hamlyn, 2004.

Kliegel, Ewald. *Crystal Wands*. Forres, Scotland: Findhorn Press, 2009.

Kynes Sandra. *Your Altar*. Woodbury, MN: Llewellyn Publications, 2007.

Linn, Denise. *Sacred Space*. London, UK: Rider, 2005.

Livoti, Dr. Carol, and Elizabeth Topp. *Vaginas: An Owner's Manual*. New York, NY: Thunder's Mouth Press, 2004.

McBride, Kami. *105 Ways To Celebrate Menstruation*. Graton, CA: Living Awareness Publications, 2004.

Medicine Eagle, Brooke. *Buffalo Woman Comes Singing*. New York, NY: Ballantine Books, 1991.

Northrup, Dr. Christiane. *The Wisdom of Menopause*. London, UK: Piatkus, 2009.

Owen, Lara. *Honoring Menstruation: A Time of Self-Renewal.* Berkeley, CA: Crossing Press (Ten Speed Press), 1998.

Roads, Michael J. *Conscious Gardening.* Forres, Scotland: Findhorn Press, 2011.

Scheffer, Mechthild. *The Encyclopedia of Bach Flower Therapy.* Rochester, VT: Healing Arts Press (Bear and Co.), 2001.

Seaward, Brian Luke. *Stand Like Mountain, Flow Like Water.* Deerfield Beach, FL: HCI Books, 1997.

Silveira, Isabel. *Quartz Crystals.* Forres, Scotland: Findhorn Press, 2008.

Vennell, David. *Healing Hands: Simple and Practical Reflexology Techniques for Developing Good Health and Inner Peace.* Hants, UK: O Books (John Hunt Publishing), 2005.

Walker, Barbara. *The Women's Encyclopedia of Myth and Secrets.* San Francisco, CA: HarperSanFrancisco, 1987.

White, Ian. *Australian Bush Flower Essences.* Forres, Scotland: Findhorn Press, 1993.

Zinn, Jon Kabbat. *Wherever You Go, There You Are: Mindfulness Meditation in Everyday Life.* London, UK: Piatkus, 2004.

Endnotes

CHAPTER 3

1. Crawford, C. *Daughters of the Inquisition*. Tensed, ID: Seven Springs Press, 2004.

2. Webster's Directory.

3. Durdin-Robertson, L. *The Cult of the Goddess*. Enniscorthy, Eire: Cesara Publications, 1974.

4. "Hunter-gatherer." *New World Encyclopedia*. 2008. *www.newworldencyclopedia.org/entry/Hunter-gatherer#Structure-of-Hunter-gatherer-Societies*. Accessed on 30.8.12.

5. Walker, Barbara. *The Women's Encyclopedia of Myth and Secrets*. San Francisco, CA: HarperSanFrancisco, 1987.

6. Harvey, Graham. *Listening People, Speaking Earth: Contemporary Paganism* (Second Edition). London, UK: Hurst and Company, 2007, ppl-2.

7. Farrar, Janet and Farrar, Stewart. *The Witches' Goddess: The Feminine Principle of Divinity*. London, UK: Robert Hale, 1987, pp29-37.

8. Museum of Menstruation and Women's Health. *www.mum.org*. Accessed on 30.8.12.

CHAPTER 4

9. John R. Lee, MD. *www.johnleemd.com*. Accessed on 30.8.12.

10. "How to Obtain Natural Progesterone." The Natural Progesterone Information Service. *www.npis.info/howtoobtain.htm*. Accessed on 30.8.12.

11. Northrup, Dr. Christiane. *The Wisdom of Menopause*. London, UK: Piatkus, 2009, pp241-243.

12. Livoti, Dr. Carol, and Elizabeth Topp. *Vaginas: An Owner's Manual*. New York, NY: Thunder's Mouth Press, 2004.

CHAPTER 5

13. The National Institute of Medical Herbalists. *www.nimh.org.uk*. Accessed on 30.8.12.

CHAPTER 6

14. The Bach Centre. www.bachcentre.com. Accessed on 30.8.12.

15. Australian Bush Flower Essences (ABFE). *www.ausflowers.com. au*. Accessed on 30.8.12.

CHAPTER 7

16. Jacobson, E. *Progressive Relaxation.* Chicago, IL: University of Chicago Press, 1938.

CHAPTER 9

17. *www.newgrange.com*. This site includes information on how white quartz might have been used in the mound or "cairn." Accessed on 30.8.12.

18. Vogel Crystals. *www.vogelcrystals.net/index.htm*. Accessed on 30.8.12.

CHAPTER 10

19. "History: Dr William H Fitzgerald MD." Modern Institute of Reflexology. *www.reflexologyinstitute.com/reflex_fitzgerald.php*. Accessed on 30.8.12.

20. "History of Reflexology." International Institute of Reflexology. *www.reflexology-usa.net/history.htm*. Accessed on 30.8.12.

Further Laurel Alexander titles

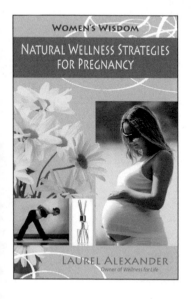 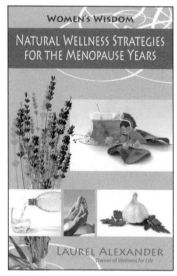

Women's Wisdom:
Natural Wellness Strategies for Pregnancy

This book on natural pregnancy offers a broad range of remedies women can use to ease and enhance their journey.

978-1-84409-585-8

Women's Wisdom:
Natural Wellness Strategies for the Menopause Years

Celebrating a reconnection with natural life cycles, thought-provoking suggestions are explored for envisioning this profound change as an important rite of passage in a woman's life.

978-1-84409-566-7

F I N D H O R N   P R E S S

Life-Changing Books

For a complete catalogue,
please contact:

Findhorn Press Ltd
117-121 High Street,
Forres IV36 1AB,
Scotland, UK

t +44 (0)1309 690582
f +44 (0)131 777 2711
e info@findhornpress.com

or consult our catalogue online
(with secure order facility) on
www.findhornpress.com

For information on the Findhorn Foundation:
www.findhorn.org